PLANT-BASED
KETO

How to cleanse your body, reduce inflammation, cholesterol and diabetes through ketogenic diet.

Low-carb vegetarian diet plan to lose weight quickly with 30 tasty veg keto recipes.

LARA RUSH

Table of Contents

FOREWORD

I must say that it is my utmost pleasure to invite you to read this book as it takes us through the path of attaining a healthy lifestyle. A lot of myths abound as to the effectiveness of practicing ketogenic nutritional diets, much more than a plant-based one. Truth be told, I also had doubts about the ketogenic dietary lifestyle at first. One of my fears was centered around the fact that I would feel choked, inhibited, and restricted from doing what I liked best: eating meat and sweetened foods. Then my friend came with news of the new cool. Of course, as inquisitive as I am, I wanted to hear all about it, and then, boom! She said we had to go on a ketogenic lifestyle to get on with the new cool. I had my eyebrows raised at once.

Cautiously, I started transitioning, and I must tell you, it took all of my willpower to sustain my resolve to go on with it. It was even better being two people looking out for each other. I would always say Suzanne was my health police. Of course, I had a lot of benefits to gain such as losing weight. I badly needed to lose weight as I had missed my trim figure. Besides, I am well into my adult life and plan on staying alive much younger.

Having heard of the risk factors of consuming foods like canned foods, processed foods, junks, meat, pastries, and all, I immediately set out like a hunter, restocking my pantry with mostly plant-based foods. This I did, not only with myself in mind but also with my children in mind, now that I know diabetes may be inherited. All junks were thrown into the bin and now, no matter how busy I am, I take the pain to make my food from the scratch, including fresh vegetables, whole grains, and fruits that have low-carb compositions, high fat, and moderate carbohydrate.

If I had not experienced the wonders of introducing plant-based foods into my diet, I would not be advising you to do the same. Besides, it is more risky to eat just about anything the animal kingdom has to offer.

And now, I would hate to hoard the amazing information about the plant-based ketogenic diet and all it entails.

I hope this would pique your curiosity enough to come along with me, turning every page of the book till you get to the very last word feeling refreshed and having your mind set to begin the plant-based ketogenic lifestyle.

Introduction

Nutrition is an integral part of a diet. It is one thing everyone expects to get from their meals. However, a lot of people do not think much about the quality of nutrition they get from foods. Due to the increasing number of fast food joints we have around town and the busy lives most of us live, we think there is really no time to eat healthy food, especially one made from scratch. One should ask, does good food really take more time to prepare and cost more than what we spend eating out? The answer is surely in the negative-NO!

Apart from the foods we eat at fast food joints, a lot of people have a routine of foods they consume, name it, bread, rice, twists, spaghetti, noodles, etc. These will definitely get boring with time and you are not really getting proper nutrition from them. In fact, you are being malnourished without realizing it. You really should avoid processed foods and refined carbs and sugars which are stripped of important nutrients that prevent sugar from being absorbed into the bloodstream too quickly.

In addition to this, the organs of your body such as the kidneys and liver are under double pressure, having to cleanse your body and remove impurities when you could easily save them the stress with more plant-based diets. If you do this, the overall effect tells on you, while you also get to live a quality life and possibly live longer. The truth is that the fast food that we eat are usually high in carbohydrate and fat, leading to an increase in blood sugar, cholesterol, and the possible risk of diabetes. According to the World Health Organization Fact Sheet, almost half of all deaths are attributable to high percentages of glucose found in the blood, while it is a major cause of blindness, kidney failure, heart attacks, stroke, and lower limb amputation. You tell yourself that you need only a small amount of energy to get you running all day long. While being active and on top of your game is admirable, eating good food is a priority that should never be brushed aside. Ever!

Eating good food means you have the right nutrients contained therein, so you do not have stunted growth. Now, vegetables are an essential part of a balanced diet for most people. Eating lots of them mean that half or almost half of your food is filled with them, and this in turn means that you are intentionally cutting down on carbohydrates. This is exactly what a keto vegetarian diet helps you eliminate- the excess carbohydrates. I know it is quite hard switching from your regular meals, where you do not really care about what makes it up, as far as it is yummy and fills your stomach quite well. But hey, you've got to watch out; you might just be adding some extra weight than you may really need.

Now, this book plans to reveal what a plant-based keto diet is all about, and just how to get your way into it. It also exposes you to ways by which you may optimize your health, lose weight instantly, cleanse your body, reduce inflammation, cholesterol, and all other things that come with them. I tell you, get ready for an amazing ride of your life, as you are about to read facts, tested and trusted. To put the feather in the cap, you get free recipes to go, and I tell you, they are equally tasty.

Simply relax, turn the pages and enjoy!

CHAPTER 1

Understanding Plant-Based Ketogenic Diet

For a lot of people, you are probably hearing the term 'plant-based keto' for the first time. This chapter will help you understand what it means in detail, laying a good foundation while we gradually lay solid blocks to ensure that you are all good on the subject.

In the last decade, there has been a fast-rising index in the number of people diagnosed with obesity, hypertension, and heart diseases in the world. This, in turn, may lead to a case that is more complicated such as depression, psychological issues, frustration cancer, inability to sleep, weight loss, and so on. These and more have been found to have links with dietary deficiencies. This is not to scare you, but to show you that the discovery of ketogenic diets came to the limelight to combat these issues as a form of dietary intervention, and since then it has gained even more popularity. Now, what is a ketogenic diet?

A ketogenic diet is that dietary combination that is characterized by a lower level of carbohydrates, usually less than 1¾ oz per day, and a significant increase in the percentages of protein and fat. The more important thing is that the percentage of protein intake is quite lower than that of fats. Hence, protein should be moderate while fats should be high, amounting to about seventy-five percent (75%) of the daily amount of calories consumed every day. This equally means that your protein intake should probably not exceed twenty percent (20%) of the total amount of calories you take in a day. The sources of foods that are high in fat and are good for a keto diet are usually animal-based products such as fish, meat, butter, and so on. However, we are going to be strictly talking about plant-based keto diets, where animal-based products are excluded.

From a critical point of view, going keto on a plant-based level means you have to carefully consider your diet. Since you are avoiding meat and all animal products, there are three essential macro nutrients that you have to take into consideration: carbs, protein, and healthy fats. Some of the meats you get in stores and markets may contribute to high carbs, so you have to be careful about them. Hence, you may want to consider other sources of healthy fats like seeds, oils, and nuts.

A keto diet enables the body to produce what is known as ketones in the liver. The liver in turn uses the ketones to generate energy. The reality is that when a person continually has a high intake of carbohydrates, a chemical reaction goes on in the body. It seems like a bell chiming, and you know what? The body then produces what is known as insulin and glucose. I am sure you must have heard of these two at one point or the other. Now, insulin does a great job of breaking down and processing the glucose you have in your blood. On the other hand, glucose is a form of energy that your body requires to function. It is in this case, a primary form of energy. When this happens, the fats which are not needed are stored, and then you begin to add weight.

It is quite obvious that you need to do something about the carbs you take, and you must do it quite fast. The moment you take immediate action, your body is caused to go into a state known as 'ketosis'. In further explanation, ketosis is a process whereby the body produces what is known as ketones, to help break up the fats which are saved up in the liver.

Basically, the aim of the ketogenic diet is to regulate the metabolism that takes place in the body, changing the main source of energy the body uses as fuel from glucose to ketone and fats. This way, the sugar level in the blood is greatly reduced, and you have no fear of an impending risk of diabetes, hypertension, or high blood pressure. When you weigh the pros and cons between glucose as a source of energy and ketones, studies reveal that ketones are cleaner burning, with a lower number of reactive oxygen, they are less inflammatory and more efficient energy givers.

According to Abbey Sharp, R.D., "ketosis has been shown to help promote weight loss because it helps suppress your hunger hormones and therefore your appetite, while also promoting substantial water loss to reduce bloating." This is the reason why you must go low on carbs if you want to lose any weight or maintain your trim body. The only way to get this done is to opt for a plant-based ketogenic lifestyle.

Plant-based keto is quite a challenge to a lot of people because you are inhibited from eating just anything. You feel restricted or grounded and may experience some form of constipation because your body is re-adjusting and trying to obtain more fiber from eating very low carb and high fat, but then it is not an impossible feat. It may also be a complete change in the lifestyle of some people and take some time to get used to. Remember that you have a goal you are striving to achieve, and at the end of it all it pays off and you only have yourself to thank. All you have to do is put on your creative gear and get started with recipes, cookbooks, and plant-based products like nuts, olives, coconut oil, avocados, and much more that we would be revealing to you as you read on. Sharon Palmer, R.D.N, already emphasized the difference between a typical vegetarian diet and a traditional keto diet when she says that "the essence of a vegetarian diet is healthful carbohydrates, and keto diets are very low in carbs". This means the vegetarian diet and keto diets are not the same. And depending on how devoted you are to a vegetarian diet, all animal products should be avoided since they are the main sources of protein that a typical ketogenic diet promotes, while many plant-based proteinous foods have a high carbohydrate percentage. An example of this is beans, so it is a no-go area.

From what we have been trying to discuss, the good news is that there is actually a way around the traditional keto diet and a typical vegetarian diet; which means that there must be a way to include a lot of vegetables that are low in carbohydrates but have higher fat compositions. Vegetarians that are on a keto diet run the risk of being low on some vitamins and minerals such as iron, fatty acids, vitamin B12, zinc, calcium, vitamin D, magnesium, and some other vital nutrients. So Palmer recommends that whole foods are a good area to focus on because they will help to ensure that you are following a good nutritional path, being slow digesting carbs which also play the role of maintaining sugar level. These may be found in fruits such as avocados, blueberries, apples, soy, tomatoes, leafy green vegetables, and legumes.

Research has shown that a plant-based ketogenic diet has a profound effect on improving the effectiveness, health, and total well-being of a person. In the long run, it reflects in easing the body of its stress, reducing the workaholic lifestyle the liver and kidneys are subjected to, regulating the sugar level in the blood, reducing heart problems and other cardiovascular diseases, as well as reducing inflammation and obesity. In the words of a nutritionist, Cassidy Payne, "a classic ketogenic diet would consist of higher fat, low-carbohydrate foods like seafood, cheese, meat, eggs, and oils as well as non-starchy vegetables, nuts, seeds, and berries"- the latter of which contain plenty fiber which is super important on a low carbohydrate diet...someone following a ketogenic, plant-based diet would focus on non-starchy vegetables such as courgette, kale, cauliflower, and mushrooms as well as fatty ones like avocados and olives. Other foods include nuts, seeds, berries, oils and perhaps some processed foods like vegan meats made from soy, unsweetened dairy alternatives made from ingredients like soy protein and coconut, and maybe sweeteners such as stevia...".

She further went on to say that "if you follow this kind of plan, particularly during exercise, you may burn higher amounts of fat. It has been associated with an expedited rate of weight loss compared to other diets. This is largely due to the initial loss of water when your liver stores of carbohydrates are used within the first few days, although, this can also result in a higher risk of dehydration. Fat loss is largely dependent on your energy intake, dietary composition, and glycaemic index, as well as the type and frequency of exercise you are doing, not forgetting the influence your genetic makeup and age also have on your metabolic rate. Whilst there is no one size fits all, some individuals have found greater success with fat or weight loss, particularly when switching from a diet heavy in processed foods to one rich in whole, plant-based foods." Indeed, the benefits which you stand to gain by opting for a plant-based ketogenic diet abound, so why not be generous with your body in this sense and marvel at the outcome?

According to the research which was given in the journal Diabetes & Metabolic Syndrome; Clinical Research & Reviews, keto diets are very instrumental in speeding up the rate at which a person may lose weight, since it burns fat approximately ten times, compared to the rate at which other diets burn fat. However, do you know that some vegetarians may still be overweight? This may happen when they rely on fruits and vegetables which are high in carbohydrates and deficient in fat. Meanwhile, a plant-based keto diet emphasizes that the percentage of carbs you should have in your meal should not exceed five to ten percent (5%-10%). If you are not sure of how to go about this, it is usually advisable to check with a nutritionist who will be a better guide for you.

Another nutritionist of importance is Adam Stansbury, who once said that "we know many plant foods come with carbohydrates, so you need to focus your intake of vegetables on low carbohydrate veg, such as green leafy and cruciferous vegetables. The keto diet is similar to the Atkins diet in that it encourages a large volume of dietary fat to make up the daily calorie intake and encourage ketosis, but the Atkins diet was not concerned with the quality of the fat or food source. The keto diet does focus more on quality foods and sources of dietary fat but still uses the same mechanism of ketosis in the body. For true ketosis to be triggered, you must eat a very low amount of carbohydrates, approximately five to ten percent of your daily calorie intake. A standard keto macronutrient split could be fat seventy percent, protein twenty percent, and carbohydrates ten percent (maybe going as low as five percent carbohydrates)."

Plant-based keto is highly beneficial in the sense that it has an inherent anti-inflammatory nature, excellent in its role of excluding sugar and gluten to ease the pressure on your digestive system which is already working overtime. Hence, to combat challenges that you may face while switching to plant-based keto, you may take multivitamins and nuts.

CHAPTER 2

Why Plant-Based Ketogenic Diet?

Originally, ketogenic diets were developed to treat epilepsy. This went as far back as the year 1924. However, ketogenic diets seem to be gaining prominence in the twenty-first century, to give solutions to weight loss, inflammation, diabetes, and other known issues. It is important to state that ketogenic diets may come in different forms such as the standard ketogenic diet (SKD), cyclical ketogenic diet (CKD), Targeted ketogenic diet (TKD), and high protein ketogenic diet (HPKD).

The Standard ketogenic diet is a diet that constitutes a very low carbohydrate with moderate protein and high fat composition. Almost everyone is familiar with what a standard ketogenic diet is since it is very good for therapeutic ketosis and weight loss. This being the case, I think it is paramount to enlighten you on the other types of keto diets.

The cyclical ketogenic diet involves periods of higher carbohydrates in between the ketogenic diet cycles. For instance, you may have five ketogenic days followed by two high carbohydrate days as a cycle. The targeted ketogenic diet involves an extra carbohydrate composition during the periods of intensive physical workout, while the high-protein ketogenic diet includes more protein ration around sixty percent (60%) fat, thirty-five percent (35%) protein, and five percent (5%) carbohydrates. The cyclical keto diet is simply a slight alteration of the standard keto diet. If you have a standard keto diet for most days of the week, say five to six days, you have to refeed immediately on high-carb diets such as oats, beans, and sweet potatoes for about one to two days. This is done to restore the glucose which your body has lost.

If you have also ever heard of 'carb cycling', then you know that it is related to cyclical keto, although they are entirely different. Carb cycling simply involves you reducing the amount of carbs you feed on for a number of days in a week while also increasing the intake of other nutrients. It performs some of the functions of the cyclical keto diet such as improvement of performance and bodybuilding. It is believed that a cyclical keto diet strategically raises insulin levels on some days to build your muscles, while it decreases the risk of consumers having flu, fatigue, headache, nausea, irritability, and so on. The major difference between the two is that carb cycling does not eventually induce the body to reach ketosis.

On the other hand, there are some side effects that the cyclical keto diet poses. For instance, you may experience some weight gain in the midst of transitioning. Basically, when you consume foods that are high in carbohydrates, much more water is retained in the body system, which leads to weight gain. I bet this was not what you bargained for when choosing it, but it is a potential risk to your weight loss goal.

Looking into what a targeted ketogenic diet entails reveals that the only variation it has with the standard keto diet is the timing of carb consumption, while it also shares the advantage of optimizing performance. Indeed, its benefits abound. Some of them are lowering the level of insulin, decreasing the risk of inflammation, having a positive effect on the body and mind, especially for those having cancer, and controlling the hunger hormone known as ghrelin, leading to a potential weight loss. Studies have shown that the targeted keto diet falls somewhere in between the standard keto diet and the cyclical keto diet. Essentially, it works for people who have their glycogen level depleted, and are into rigorous exercises or sports. Hence, consuming the right amount of carbs, ranging from ½ oz to 1¾ oz around the time of your workout, is a huge benefit. That is exactly why it is 'targeted'. However, there is a risk that targeted keto poses, and it is such that it may block you out of the ketosis cycle. This is because you consume lots of carbs at a specific time, leading to an increase in the sugar level in your blood and this subsequently reduces the amount of ketone produced in your body system. Remember we mentioned earlier that ketones are better energy producers, anti-inflammatory, and cleaner than glucose.

Now considering the last of the types of keto diets, which is the high protein keto diet. Proteins have been found to help the body in the process of building bones, skin care, and muscle tone building. In a high protein keto diet, the percentage of proteins should be higher than carbs and should make about thirty percent (30%) of calories, sixty-five percent (65%) of fats, and five percent (5%) of carbs. Nuts and seeds are good sources of protein. If you notice that you are also deficient in protein and need muscle building and full hair, this may be a good choice for you, but if you are undergoing therapy, it is advisable to stay away from high protein foods. Also, care has to be taken with the consumption of protein, as a build-up may lead to kidney issues. Much protein has also been found to reduce the amount of ketones in the blood, thereby reducing your better energy booster.

According to the Indian Journal of Medicine, the standard ketogenic diet (SKD) and high protein ketogenic diet (HPKD) have been used extensively and have been around longer than the other types. The cyclical and targeted ketogenic diets are recent additions and are mostly used by people who want to build their bodies and muscles, such as athletes. Research has shown that athletes who had a periodic intake of high carbs showed a tremendous improvement in their performance compared to the other types of keto diets.

Having considered the pros and cons of all the types of ketogenic diets and having had background knowledge of them all, we will delve into the plant-based keto diet and why it is the best choice for you.

Why should your diets be plant-based? What are the benefits? Are the sources easily accessible? How can you maintain your plant-based diet without getting bored? These and more are explained below.

A plant-based diet simply means there is an inclusion of vegetables, fruits, or some grains in your food composition. It involves replacing the animal-based products you eat with the ration of vegetables. So basically, any food substance which has a high composition of plant, has a reduced level of carbs, and induces your body to ketosis, is a proper plant-based diet.

Are you unsure as to the types of plant-based keto diets? Let us take a look at something interesting.

Some diets are entirely plant-based in their compositions. Some of these include a typical vegan meal. It is strictly veggies, with zero amount of animal-based products. Eggs and dairy products are also excluded from these diets. Hence, there are lacto-vegetarians (people who consume dairy products), pescatarians (people who feed mainly on plants, eggs, dairy products, and seafood), ovo-vegetarians (people who feed on eggs but never dairy products), flexitarians (people who take plant-based diets but also include a moderate amount of meat and other animal-based products). All these are variations of vegetarians. Indeed, studies reveal that about 40% of Americans are striving to include plant-based products in their diets. This corresponds with an increase in the amount of groceries that are being purchased daily by Americans.

As a person who wants to transition into a plant-based keto diet, you have to condition your mind to a few facts. One of these is that you have to keep your carbohydrate intake very low. There exist some kinds of vegetables which are high in carbs, so you have to be careful when choosing your veggies. At the end of this book, you will find enough ways to pick your veggies to benefit you and still get you into ketosis. In addition, you may want to try being a variant of one of the vegetarian types as spelled out above, in your transitioning process. This is because they give you the advantage of also trying out a variety of protein sources, just like the flexitarians.

Protein is a nutrient that is highly important in a person's diet. It is split into smaller bits known as amino acids to help you with healthy skin, tissue building, hormonal secretion, and balance. Some of the functions it performs are protecting the health of your heart, strengthening white blood cells and your overall immune system, and boosting your physical energy. In relation to this, a plant-based diet has a proper amount of protein to optimize your health potential.

If you are looking to commence plant-based dietary nutrition, the first step to take is to make up your mind as to which of the options to go with. As spelled out above, you could choose to be a standard vegetarian, a flexitarian, a lacto-vegetarian, an ovo-vegetarian, or a pescatarian. It means you are mentally conditioning yourself, preparing your mind to go with it. There is a need to gradually ease yourself into it. Ask yourself basic questions like if you can do without some foods, meats, fish, nuts, or oils even in the worst situations. If there is no way you can let go, then it would be better not to start at all. Also, making a choice would help you in its sustainability, especially if you have goals of weight loss or health maintenance and optimization.

Energy Sustenance

An advantage that is evident in consuming plant-based products is that the amount of clean energy-giving ketones your body is able to produce increases. This means you are enhancing the natural process of your body getting into ketosis, a metabolic process that would aid the functioning of vital organs like the kidneys and the liver. Remember that your carbs must be kept low too if you want to get into ketosis. How do you get this done? You may choose veggies that are low in carbs. These include kale, broccoli, cucumber, celery, leafy green veggies, and so on. At least one of them should be included in your meals, and you could get creative with a combination of them too.

Diabetes Control

Research reveals that consuming lots of veggies, fruits and grains helps a lot in reducing the risks of cancer and other diseases. This is because plants have a special ingredient known as phytochemicals, and these have been discovered to aggressively tackle cancerous cells. Compare this to eating red meat, a potential trigger of cancer. In addition to this, a vegan diet reduces the risk of diabetes. Diabetes is essentially a condition that inhibits the body's ability to process glucose. You know, when you take food into your body system, it undergoes a process of breaking down into smaller components. Enzymes and chemicals work on them to do this. It has been recorded that over thirty percent (30%) of the total population of people living in the United States are living with diabetes, which may either be Type 1, Type 2, or gestational diabetes. Studies have also shown that diabetes may be inherited, especially by people who have a family history of high cholesterol or diabetes. This may lead to so much more complications if care is not taken. The complications may include heart attack, chest pain, heart diseases, and stroke. People who eat more plant-based foods are insulin sensitive, a vital part of maintaining the sugar level in the blood. While no cure has yet been found for diabetes, proper management may be followed effectively.

As a matter of fact, meat eaters have a double risk of having diabetes as vegans, lacto-vegetarians, and ovo-vegetarians. Seeing this, you might want to consider including more plant-based products in your meals.

Vegetables and fruits, as you have found out, have good vitamins, minerals, and fiber contents, which are good for metabolism, prevent heart disease and diabetes, and also good for your health in general. They not only aim at improving the way your body controls sugar in the blood but also reduce blood pressure and control cholesterol. They are anti-inflammatory and help to build your arteries. This means your heart becomes healthier and you have a quality life span.

Better Mental Health

Having a sustainable vegetarian life will require much more commitment than you can ever imagine but at the end of it all, your body gets the right amount of macronutrients needed to keep you going. Your mental health also enjoys lots of benefits from eating plant-based foods. Stress management is an integral aspect of mental health, and may be traced to your diet which in turn takes a toll on your overall body functions. When your diet is not right, you tend to be at your lowest capacity. Wonder why some people break down suddenly? It is because they are overwhelmed by too much stress, there is stress on their body systems, they are not feeding well, their emotions (hormones) are at an all-time low, and it affects their relations with people too. Switching to a plant-based diet thus, is the easy way out for you because your hormones become more balanced, you are able to sleep better, your mental performance is optimized, you have better vision, your head is clearer and you can easily think things through, confusion is reduced, you get a new shine to your skin, and you are essentially at your best.

Depression is a mental issue that is continually on the rise globally. In fact, it has been found to affect even more women compared to men. Considering the data collected by the National Health and Nutrition

Examination Survey in America between the periods of 1988 and 1994, severe depression was found to be dominant in obese women. The studies further reveal that factors that trigger depression include cultural, social, and psychological factors and the stigma attached is intricately bound with the self-esteem of these people, ultimately leading to their possible suicide. Hence, everyone seems to go about in a frenzy looking for fast means of losing weight. This is because they have been tagged with the word "fat". The world seems to scorn overweight people. In fact, entertainment shows and the media, in general, seem to adore trim bodies and flat tummies. Now, ask me why depression would not definitely set in. Well, a number of women have attached their self-image to what they see on TV, or their TV stars, models, and all other people. They just want to be perfect no matter what it costs, even if it has to do with extremes.

For this reason, the plant-based ketogenic diet offers an easy and simple way to lose weight. It simply involves being cautious about your diet, eating low carbs, high fat and moderate protein. Really, no one needs to go through the pains of depression as a result of their body size and weight.

Other uses of a plant-based ketogenic diet for mental health include the reduced risk of brain cancer, Parkinson's disease, autism, pain, lateral sclerosis, and sleep disorders. So you see, your mental health is reliant on your diet.

Epilepsy Control

Eating a plant-based nutritional diet is not restricted to men or women alone. Children may also be given. From a very young period of their lives, they need protein and other essential nutrients which serve as building blocks in their formative years. These nutrients can have a significant effect on reducing their risk of using glasses. Since keto was originally discovered to combat epilepsy which is difficult to control, children are saved from seizures with a ketogenic diet of a ratio 4:1 in terms of weight of fat to carbohydrates and proteins. Let us take a practical look at how epilepsy may be avoided.

Epilepsy is a neurological disorder that affects at least 50 million people around the world. It is recognized by multiple seizures and a disruption of the normal functioning of the brain. Subsequently, such a person having epilepsy loses consciousness. You will recall that a ketogenic diet is mainly composed of low carbs, high fat and the right amount of protein, isn't it? Now, what happens with these is that the diet induces the body to burn fat, replacing the function of carbohydrates in this sense. Naturally, carbohydrates in food are converted to glucose and circulated in the bloodstream to give energy and enhance the function of the brain. On the other hand, with the low quantity of carbohydrates in the diet, the liver is triggered to perform some special function which is to convert fat into fatty acids and ketones. This ketone is then circulated in the body to replace glucose as an energy-giving body, hence, ketosis. Finally, the metabolic state and function of ketosis is that which reduces the frequency of epileptic seizures.

As far back as 1994, Charlie Abrahams, a two-year-old son of the popular Hollywood producer suffered from epilepsy, a condition that apparently could not be controlled by drugs and alternative therapies. One day, his father stumbled on the miraculous ketogenic diet which transformed Charlie's life and restored his health to normalcy. Just this brought explosive research to keto and it is widely practiced by people today.

Now, it was discovered that when children suffering from epileptic seizures tried out ketogenic diets, the frequency of the crisis was reduced by fifty percent (50%) in the least. This is because of its therapeutic nature which needs just the right amount of protein for the growth and repair of tissues with enough calories for proper maintenance of the correct weight and height of the child. It was even found out that the effect of this diet persisted even when the diet was no longer continued. In fact, children who tried keto respond faster to treatment than those who tried alternative forms of diets. Hence, to achieve this, there is a need to avoid foods that are high in carbs such as bread, pasta, sugar, some grains, and starchy fruits or vegetables.

Hopefully, you can evidently see that the benefits of having a plant-based keto diet are numerous. If you have any more questions, it would be advisable to consult your nutritionist or a medical doctor.

CHAPTER 3

Getting Trim With Veggies

Welcome to a new page, where you will learn how to effectively combine foods, essentially vegetables to help you lose weight. Scientifically speaking, plant-based keto diets have been found to produce better results in the aspect of burning fat, compared to other diets with high carbs in them. Hence, they provide evident reasons to be chosen over all other kinds of diets.

Over the years, obesity has posed a great headache for most people and the search for ways to slim down with immediacy has been on for ages. Let us examine some facts and challenges facing obese people. The World Health Organization seems to be in agreement with the National Heart, Lung, and Blood Institute on what it means to be overweight. They conclude that being overweight is based on the body mass index, otherwise known as the BMI. It simply refers to the value you get by dividing your weight by the square of your height. The value lets you know if you are underweight, normal weight, overweight or obese, based on your muscle, fat, bones, and height. Usually, for adults, the healthy BMI is between 18.9 and 24.9. Hence, the moment you exceed this range, you are on the obese side. While some women easily notice that they have gained some pounds by the thickness around their waist circumference, it is preferable to check your BMI for the proper value.

Most people, especially women, have their self-image attached to the way they look. So each time they look at themselves in the mirror, they are critical and sad. It has become a big issue for them, and they are searching for all means to eliminate it. When this is the case, sometimes, their morale is low, and it is even worse when their partners or husbands begin to complain about fat in some places. They begin to wonder where all the trim body disappeared to. But then, it doesn't just appear overnight.

One of the numerous reasons why you cannot reach your desired trimness is your unhealthy diet. Eating overly spiced foods, and adding extra salt to food can be detrimental to your body system. In fact. Let me also add that foods that are deficient in potassium ultimately cause water retention in the body, while you also stand the risk of high blood pressure. But what foods contain the proper potassium content your body needs? Have you considered eating more plant-based foods and leafy greens? They contain just the right amount of potassium composition needed by your body.

Eating good food and staying healthy seem to have a whole lot of rules for us, and you can bet that we as humans never love to be restricted by rules. In fact, having to condition our body systems can be worse; it revolts and the first thing that comes to our minds is to stop the nutritious but challenging diet. You begin to question how you got here in the first place and before you know it, you have resolved to damn all the consequences of being obese.

For a lot of people who seem to be extremely busy, you would notice that you do not have time to cook, so you eat almost any food without caring to know what makes it up. In the case of mothers who have so many children to look after, you would notice that every other person comes first and you mostly forget to look after yourself in terms of paying attention to your body. This way, obesity comes knocking, opens the door boldly, and makes itself comfortable without so much as a call of invitation from you. Now, on the very first day of every year, your New Year's Resolution, I mean the very first one on the list, is to lose weight and even more weight.

Endocrine glands also have contributions to obesity, especially in women whose bodies seem to always act funny when their menstrual cycles come calling. Hormones like estrogen and progesterone are trickery. During menstrual cycles, the hormonal level varies from woman to woman. During the course of it all, you may discover that you feel bloated due to water retention. But where does the water disappear after the period? Mysterious, isn't it?

This makes up pretty much the same story for pregnant women and some women who may experience hormonal fluctuation as a result of the use of contraceptives. Now, if the bloating persists, it is very important for you to consult a doctor. But I am sure that one of the questions you would be asked is if you are observing a proper diet. Have no fears, eating proper plant-based foods is the right antidote to obesity or weight gain. So, how do you go about shedding the excess fat? Here are some tips for you:

- Have a red alert on processed foods: it is quite important to learn to reduce the amount of processed foods you consume. For a transition into a plant-based diet, it is also advisable to gradually ease yourself into it. This way, you are not shocking your body organs, but allowing them to easily accept the changes that are being introduced into the system. More salads and fruits that are low in carbs are sure to play the role perfectly. All animal-based products in your food can be replaced with plant-based substitutes like mushrooms, kale, and cauliflower. Also try to build your food from scratch yourself, rather than eating processed foods from restaurants and fast food joints.

In addition to this, most packaged foods are high in flour, sugar, salt, refined oils, saturated fats, and too much amino acids, so be careful to look out for these.

- Restock your pantry: it is increasingly easy to incorporate plant-based products into your food. Our markets offer a wider range of plant-based foods than there ever were. Now, you would find kale chips and dairy-free milk in grocery stores, and they look good too. All that you have to do is to replace all animal-based products with plant-based foods, and since there is a lot of creativity by producers of foods now, you can enjoy yourself as you browse the grocery stores and supermarkets in your search of brand new options to match your new lifestyle. Snacks as well as whole foods are now made with plant-based compositions, so for a quick snack at work, for your children, at picnics, or for breakfast, plant-based foods can rock.
- Consider the nutrient composition of packaged foods: as much as there are interestingly new products in the markets today, not all of

them have the right health composition for your new plant-based diets. For a proper plant-based keto diet, have it at the back of your mind that you are in search of low carbs, high fat, and moderate protein composition. In plant-based keto foods, you find low carbs and amino acids in different proportions. So there is plenty of protein in them to meet your daily requirements. According to a well-known nutritionist, "as long as you are eating enough calories to sustain yourself and are focusing on whole foods instead of refined foods, it would be impossible to become deficient in protein." You may be interested in considering plant-based low-carb proteins like rice protein produced from sprouted brown rice and hemp seeds rich in magnesium, potassium, fiber, and fatty acids. Broccoli, cucumber, onion, lettuce, celery stalks, avocado, eggplants, and kale are great additions to your plant-based ketogenic diets.

- Find alternatives: finding substitutes for your favorite but unhealthy foods can be quite an uninteresting task. But hey, you know you want to slim down, and you want it real bad. So just shut your eyes to the bad and find fun ways to make up for them. Supplements such as vitamin B12, vitamin A, vitamin B3 & B6, iron, and iodine are fantastic components of plant-based foods. You may wish to substitute milk with almond and unsweetened milk, cheese with avocado, cream in your coffee with coconut cream, and so on.

- Make nuts and seeds eating your best friend: Nuts like hazelnuts and almonds have been discovered to contain lots of minerals and vitamins but you have to avoid eating cashew nuts and pistachios; this is because they contain high carbs. Chia seeds, pumpkin seeds, sesame seeds, and sunflower seeds have also been found to be a pleasant addition to your plant-based diet since they have about ½ to 1 oz of protein.

- Use healthy oils: oils are a good source of fat that is needed for a healthy plant-based keto diet. They are good sources of unsaturated fats to help your heart maintain a healthy state. But where do you find them? They are found in oils such as olive oil, coconut oils, almonds, and avocado oil, while you completely exclude vegetable seed oils like sunflower seed oil, corn oil, soy oil, and canola. This is because vegetable oils are highly processed and contain a fatty acid content known as omega-6 fatty acid which is high in composition, and may expose you to the possible risk of inflammation. These should replace butter in your diet. Coconut oil is just the ideal choice for desserts, baking, and cooking while olive oil has a very nice fragrance and flavor to make your food inviting. Additional virgin olive oil proves an even more beautiful addition to your dressings and keto-vegan salads. On the other hand, choosing avocado oil means you are choosing a healthy mono-saturated oil, an equally nice oil suitable for your plant-based meals.

- Spice up your menu: switching to a whole new diet can be very boring, as expected. But if you are to stay in the game, you have to find your way around it, and the only way to go about it is to try fun and creative ways of spicing up your menu. Do not restrict yourself to one or two recipes when there is a whole new world of plant-based foods to explore. You may try adding some veggies to your breakfast, plant-based chips as light snacks, and fruits in your dessert combination. Smoothies can also be spiced up with chocolate almond too. Hmmm! Heavenly!

There is something of a fact to keep to heart in the Journal of General Internal Medicine and I would love to share this with you. It says that people who eat more plant-based foods and vegetables are well on their way to losing the extra fat they have on them, compared to those who eat meat. In fact, over a thousand people were found to lose an approximate value of four pounds on average, compared to their counterparts on an 18-week course. Meat eaters usually have more gas retained in them, leading to bloating and uneasiness but eating vegetables, whole grains, and plant-based foods makes you feel lighter, stronger and energized, thanks to the right amount of calories and nutrients they contain. Consider eating sandwiches with veggies, mustard-crusted tofu with sweet potato or kale, cauliflower steaks, apricots, carrots, zucchini, peanuts, lentils, and so on. So, if you have chosen to go keto with plant-based diets, you are on the right path. You will soon discover significant changes to keep you happy in your entire lifetime.

Intermittent Fasting Versus Plant-Based Keto

If you were to choose between healthy ketogenic diets and fasting, which one would you opt for? Would you rather consider combining the two? These two issues seem to be making headlines in the health sector; here is what you need to know about fasting...

In France, as far back as 1911, there existed about twenty patients having epileptic fits. Doctors resolved to achieve detoxification through an alteration in the patients' diets. How did they manage to pull this through? They simply combined fasting and purging with veggie diets of low-calorie compositions. Did this pay off? It sure did! Those who were able to stick to this alteration had their mental health improved tremendously, and they totally dumped prescriptions since they had a negative effect of dulling their minds. Interestingly in those days, while a royal doc believed that it would be great to completely place epileptic patients on a merciless round of fasting with rationed food, another was of the opinion that milder cases can be dealt with, through intermittent fasting. Later in the years, there was an adoption of the fasting therapy while balancing it with a sugar and starch-free diet.

From the above illustration, deductions can be made as to what it means to have an intermittent fasting period. Let me spell it out. Intermittent fasting simply entails the process you have to go through reducing the amount of calorie consumption (otherwise known as fasting) and eating normal food. You may as well call it a rotation of both within specific periods of time. Let us have a quick look at the types of intermittent fasting in existence:

- Fasting two days a week: this type of fasting has otherwise been tagged the "5:2 diet". Why is this case? Simply, it involves eating about five hundred (500) to six hundred (600) calories for only two out of seven days in the week, while you are free to eat normally for five days.
- Complete day's fast: this is the type of fasting where you don't eat any food at all for the entire day. Can you really do this without

dying? Definitely. You may as well do this once a week, so you do not have to fret about being starved to death for the whole week. Have this easier done for you by eating breakfast today, and fasting until the next breakfast, or dinner today and fasting until the next dinner.

- The Lean gains Protocol: this method of dieting or fasting means you fast for about sixteen (16) hours every day and eat normal food for only eight (8) hours. Women may do better by fasting for fifteen hours and eating for nine (9) hours.
- Fasting when you can: this method only goes for you if you feel you are not really feeling hunger pangs. It is spontaneous in nature.
- Heavy eating at night: this method of eating was popularized by Ori Hofmekler, and he interestingly termed it the "warrior diet". As funny as it sounds, it means eating nothing at all during the day, until night when you can treat yourself to a feast of whole or unprocessed foods.
- Alternate fasting: you can easily deduce from the name that it involves eating normally for a day and fasting throughout the next day.

While a lot of people have gone on a fasting adventure trying to lose some weight, other people have considered the therapeutic effects of plant-based diets. But which is more effective?

For one, intermittent fasting has been found to give some benefits, in the sense that it is also an effective method of slimming down, healthy living, and better metabolism. On the other hand, eating a plant-based diet adds nutrients to your body and you do not need to go hungry at all. Combining both of them may help you lose weight faster than if you stick to one plan or even speed up your body's inducement into ketosis. However, I would not strongly recommend practicing both at the same time if you are in a critical health condition, breastfeeding, or pregnant.

CHAPTER 4

Body Cleansing And All There Is To It

Now that you know how important making plant-based diets your nutritional choice is, I am happy to add to your excitement. This is the fact that feeding on plant-based foods helps to cleanse your body. Most of the time, body cleansing has been used synonymously with detoxification. So, we would be looking at what it means to have a body cleansing in depth.

Body cleansing or detoxification involves the processes that the body goes through in order to evacuate all impurities and toxins that have prospective harmful effects on the overall well-being of a person. Dieting or fasting has been found to be a very effective means of eliminating all these toxins. Over the years, detoxification has evolved to place itself dominantly in the medical world, as a form of an alternative method of medicine, and to add to this, it is quite prominent in its practice. Now, to satisfy your curiosity about what kinds of impurities the body removes, I'll answer by stating them- processed foods, preservatives, flavors, food sweeteners and so much more.

Let me tell you something, and it is that our bodies have a way of naturally cleaning up, thanks to the liver and kidneys which work in sync to ensure that toxins are eliminated through the bloodstream and disposed of. In today's market, there are just enough processed foods with preservatives we consume. These are made with chemicals, which is why they have expiry dates. We continually eat foods from cans and boxes so much as a care in the world sometimes, just to ease the hunger pangs. Wait a minute! You may just be doing yourself more harm than good. According to the popular detox diet, toxins include heavy metals, pollutants, and chemicals, apart from processed foods while ways of eliminating such have been listed to include the use of drugs, herbal tea, diuretics, and so on.

The chemicals and preservatives we consume introduce toxins into our body systems, thereby gradually making us unhealthy. The more we consume such canned foods, the more we place much more work in the hands of our kidneys and liver which begin to get stressed out and suddenly fail. I am sure you do not want this to happen; well, neither does a plant-based diet.

Why Should You Cleanse Your System?

1. Energy optimization: biology reveals to us that one of the health benefits of detoxing is to boost energy. Digestion is not as simple as you may think. It goes beyond putting food in your mouth and feeling it in your tummy. So free up some space in you by cleansing. The kidneys and livers, when cleansed, are at their best. But if you do not cleanse them, they are overworked and become slow.

2. Mental soundness: mental health is the direct effect of the total well-being of the body. According to research, cortisol is a hormone that is produced when the body is overworked. These may affect the proper functioning of the kidneys and liver. Hence, body cleansing helps to regulate the production of the hormone cortisol. On the other hand, the body is stressed through the intake of processed foods, alcohol, and caffeine which produces a strain on your adrenaline and prevents a healthy sleeping cycle. So for a restoration of a good sleeping pattern, a boost in mental alertness, and removal of toxins from the body, a healthy diet is good for you.

3. Reduction in bloating and constipation: plant-based foods and leafy green vegetables keep the body rejuvenated and fresh. If you have a healthy diet, less water is retained in the body, and bowel movement is boosted.

How does detoxification work?

Depending on the type of cleansing to be done, it basically requires that excess fats stored in your body are released as toxins into your bloodstream, and subsequently eliminated. It would therefore be interesting to also let you know that the elimination method is not only restricted to urine or feces. Even breathing out (exhalation) does a good job of pushing out bad air, while your skin pores do their part of the job by letting out sweat which of course contains salt and other unnecessary materials. Above all, it is a way your body says, "thanks guys, but your services are not needed anywhere around here."

Proponents of body cleansing claim that detoxification helps promote healthy intestinal bacteria, great energy boosting, and commencement of weight loss. While there are still buzzing concerns about the effectiveness of detoxification, it is claimed that cleansing diets combined with intermittent fasting and restricting some foods promote good health. For instance, the use of laxatives, herbal tea, and lots of water are frequently recommended. An excellent way to eliminate toxins from the bloodstream is to include plant-based foods in your daily meals, rather than processed foods. It is really better to build your foods from scratch, there, you will know what exactly makes up your food, and you can be fresher.

Types Of Body Cleansing

It has been discovered that various organs of the body require cleansing. You obviously do not expect that litters and dirt continue to lie around your house and nothing is being done to eliminate them, or better still, why do you feel the need to have your bath daily and sometimes 2-3 times a day? Is it because it is the outer part of your body or because whatever is hidden does not require much attention? This is just the same way to sweep and scrub your body system. Tons and tons of drugs are continually produced and prescribed by the medical and pharmaceutical industries, leading to a dependence on drugs by people and also increasing the toxicity of the body. Now imagine the amount of cleaning you have to do to a dirty house. Of course, if we need our organs to function to the best of their capacity and even prolong our lives, then quality living should be the topmost choice of each and everybody on earth. Let us examine the types of cleansing needed by the necessary organs, one after the other.

- The Colon: this is the part of the large intestine which plays a big part in the digestive system. It is divided into the ascending colon, the transverse colon, the descending colon, and the sigmoid colon. The ascending colon transports waste into the transverse colon, and on it goes until the waste products get to the rectum and out through the anus. So you may as well see it as a tube assisting the intestines. As small as it may look, its function cannot be excluded in the digestion process. Hence, it reabsorbs waste products in fluids to be expelled from the body with the help of tiny finger-like networks of capillaries known as villi. These villi have both outer and inner parts. They swim in the blood and collect nutrients before distributing them into the bloodstream. The outer part is lined with epithelial cells through which toxins may enter and cause enough trouble to kill a person, coupled with the fact that everyone is different, having different levels of tolerance to toxins and chemicals acceptable by the body.

Since the colon is a part of the large intestine, its primary function is not to absorb waste; the small intestine does that quite well. So, it "reabsorbs" the impurities. This way, the water and salt balance in the body is regulated. Most of the foods we eat pass through the small intestine before the large intestine and through the colon.

The linings of our intestines are daily exposed to toxins which frequently run the risk of accumulation, otherwise known as toxic overload. Examples of daily exposure come from food, beverages (such as concentrated juice with artificial sweeteners and colorings, pasteurized milk, and soft drinks), alcohol, sugars, salts, processed foods (in flour, ice cream, desserts, genetically manipulated foods, fast foods, canned foods, hydrogenated oils and so on), polluted airs (for instance smoke, exhaust pipes, fossil fuels, benzene, molds, sprays, etc.), polluted waters (as from chlorine, arsenic, fluoride, bisphenol used in making plastic water bottles), toxins from drug chemicals (for instance aluminium, chemotherapy, mercury, synthetic hormones), parasites, worms, fungi, viruses, decomposed materials, stress, microwaves and x-rays, and all other things we do not pay attention to. When they build up, we may feel constipated and our bowel movement is affected. Studies have shown that approximately sixty percent (60%) of Americans are living with constipation and obesity due to a lack of cleansing.

Once the colon is not cleansed, it may lead to a 'leaky gut syndrome'. What does this mean? It means tiny holes are formed in the intestines due to poor nutrition, dependence on drugs, and other toxins and chemicals. Other diseases which gradually reduce the functionality of the tissues and cells found in the body (degenerative diseases) are also likely to occur.

- **The Kidneys:** the kidneys do a great job of filtering dirt out of the body. How do you know the kidneys in the human anatomy? They are two little bean-shaped organs found on either side of the spinal cord, just below the ribs. They also help to balance hormonal secretion and flush excess waste out of the body. If you are looking forward to having strong kidneys to last you a lifetime, then you have to cleanse them. Eating healthy foods is one sure way of naturally cleansing the kidneys. Supplements such as vitamin B-6 and Omega-3, and vegetables do their best too. But all in all, water is the first point of call in a kidney cleansing process. Drinking lots of water and proper nutrition prevents the advent of kidney stones or kidney failure.

- **The Liver:** the liver is a reddish-brown organ located on the right side of the body and protected by the rib cage. On either side of it are the right and left lobes which play the role of absorbing and digesting the foods we eat before filtering them into the bloodstream. The synthesis, that is, the breaking down of glucose and lipids are integral in the work of the liver in the digestion process while insulin and glucagon regulate metabolism. In essence, metabolism, coupled with good body cleansing can protect the liver from harmful drugs. The liver also secretes a substance known as bile and other forms of proteins such as fatty acids, insulin, and cholesterol that help to clot or heal wounds speedily. The liver works in sync with the kidneys in removing waste products and balancing the natural functioning of the body. Essentially, the liver extracts the waste products which are carried through the blood and transports them to the kidney which then lets them out through urine. Without cleansing the liver, the body runs the risk of several diseases and infections such as hepatitis, cancer, jaundice, fibrosis, tumor, and the like. Symptoms preceding these diseases are fatigue, palpitations of the heart, itchy skin, excreting blood with feces, yellowing of the eyes, nausea, and so on.

- **The Skin:** this is an aspect of the natural ways the body cleanses itself. Just below your skin are thousands of little tubes known as capillaries. They are filled with blood and enhance the exchange of oxygen. You also have hair follicles and pores on your skin through which oils are excreted, and sweat too. So you see, impurities are removed through the skin.

- **The Lungs:** the lungs are extremely significant to the human respiratory system. They are linked to the nose through which oxygen is breathed in and carbon dioxide is breathed out. Other organs of the body that aid respiration are the trachea, bronchi, and diaphragm. We do not need carbon dioxide in our system, that is why it is let out as a waste product. This is also a natural way the body cleanses itself. Climate change however seems to be a hindrance to pure oxygen needed to be breathed in. Why is this the case? A lot of companies and industries let out huge quantities of carbon dioxide into the air which depletes the oxygen reserve. Exhaust fumes from cars, trucks, and other vehicles also are released into the atmosphere, most of which travel in the air to affect the ozone layer. This is why efforts have been made around the world to "go green". Everyone is affected by climate change. The ice lands are beginning to disintegrate, leading to an increase in the water level of water bodies. This leads to flooding of lands and loss of lives and property. Hence, there is a constant and conscious need to grow trees, and even more trees since trees make use of the carbon dioxide we do not use while letting out oxygen. They help to purify the environment and also when we eat veggies and plant-based products, we are optimizing our health. In one word, pollution is a central factor of increasing global concern inhibiting body cleansing.

One of the disadvantages toxins may cause to our bodies is a disruption of our hormones. Without knowing it, you realize that you are cranky even when you are nowhere near your period. Remember that endocrine glands are immensely responsible for hormonal production, hence, the food we take in may help them produce just enough that we need. So if you do not feed well, you may actually be triggering them to produce more than enough or below what is needed. Without saying much more, plant-based diets are available, ready to come to your aid if only you would call them to balance things up.

How To Detoxify Your System

Apart from the natural way the body cleanses itself, every individual also has some contribution to make to enhance this. It is not as difficult as it may seem, especially for those people who are already so adapted to a particular lifestyle. So, below are some tips I hope would be helpful to you.

- **Drink more water:** I am very sure there cannot be an over-emphasizing of this. Water is simply life. It is a natural cleanser and once you make this a part of you, it would surprise you how immensely it would ease all the other organs in your system. Also, it would tell on you. Apart from it being the first thing to take to ease your thirst, it plays a grand role in balancing your body temperature, maintaining plus repairing worn-out tissues and cells, conveyance of waste products to the necessary organs involved in passing them out, hydration, aiding the digestion process and metabolism, absorbing the nutrients from foods which are needed by the body, and ultimately detoxification.

  Every day, you should drink an approximate amount of 4-6 liters of water. By increasing your water intake, your body secretes a kind of hormone known as the antidiuretic hormone. This increases the amount of urine you pass out. But this is a huge plus to you, so you do not have to get irritated with your frequent visits to the bathroom; you just helped yourself eliminate toxins.

If you are the kind of person that feels dehydrated easily, rather than opting for carbonated drinks and juices, water should be your first and most frequent point of call.

- **Stay away from sugar and extra salt:** A lot of us have sweet mouths or better still cravings for sweet things. If you are a fan of ice cream, chocolate, sweets, carbohydrates, drinks, or other junks floating around in super marts and tuck shops, then you might as well reconsider now. You do not have to experience a toothache to halt now. Sugar is broken down into glucose and fructose. While the former is metabolized by cells in the body, the latter cannot. Now, only the liver can come to your aid in metabolizing sugar through conversion into glycogen. Glycogen is the storehouse of glucose which makes the liver further break glycogen into fructose, thereby causing a fatty liver. It has been observed amongst the larger population of the world that diseases such as cancer and diabetes are a result of high sugar intake. For one, sugar is the end product of digestion of carbohydrates. This is why plant-based keto foods are good for you since they contain low carbs which end the sugar troubles.

Salt, on the other hand, tells the body to retain more fluid. Hence you have to take more water to balance the concentration of your body system in terms of fluids, and to be passed out through your urine and sweat. Apart from this, taking too much salt subsequently puts you at risk of hypertension and high blood pressure. A good way to get rid of sugar and salts is to cut your intake of processed foods. Now is the time to start making your food from scratch. It pays you better.

- **Reduce your intake of alcoholic drinks:** taking too much alcohol means extra work for your liver. If you do not do this, it would grievously affect you in the long run by causing inflammation and tissue scarring. Besides, your heart condition is also at risk. Having too much alcohol in the body exerts more pressure on the liver in processing it. This happens when acetaldehyde, a chemical substance, is produced by the liver every time alcohol is present in the blood. This chemical has a direct effect on the linings of your stomach and also invites a buildup of fat in the liver. All these combined may in turn affect the brain. The same goes for an excessive lifestyle of smoking. These have a direct effect on the lungs and limit the natural cleansing of the body, just as they may also affect the heart.

- **Replace processed foods with plant-based foods:** Processed foods cause us more harm than good. This is because they have a high amount of additives. To cleanse the body, caution has to be taken. This is why you should cut down on them and switch to plant-based diets that are healthier, fresher, and more nutritious. Your life span also beams more promises by staying healthy. For instance, you may try eating veggies that are rich in potassium and sulphur, such as cauliflower. These help to balance out the hormones while also expelling the toxins from the body system.

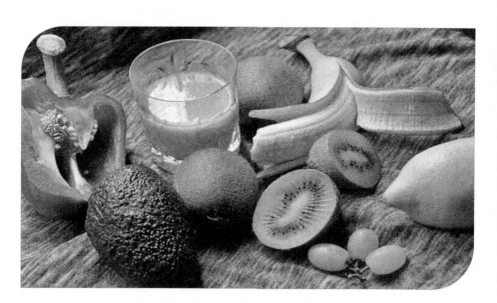

Fine Foods To Help You Out

Garlic: garlic helps to flush out toxins from the body. This is because they contain compounds such as sulphur, allicin, and other enzymes to help organs of the body. It has been found to treat fungal skin infections, acne, stretch marks, whitehead removal, and spots, and serves as an anti-aging ingredient.

Avocado: glutathione-producing compounds may be found in avocados, preventing an accumulation of toxic materials in organs such as the kidney and liver. They are a healthy source of fat to help in your plant-based keto diet.

Tumeric: this is a fine spice that helps to promote the production of bile in the liver. It also helps to reduce inflammation, regenerate cells in the body, and cleanse the internal organs of the body.

Spinach: this is a leafy green vegetable that stimulates the growth of cells and contains a nutrient known as beta carotene. This is perfect for your plant-based keto diet.

Beetroot juice: obtained from beets, the body gains vital vitamins and minerals such as fiber, potassium, folic acid, magnesium, and vitamins A, B, and C. For a fine recipe of beetroot juice, get apples, kale, carrots, lemon, and ginger to go with it.

Brussels sprouts: combined with cabbage and broccoli, you can never be wrong. Brussels sprouts are high in sulfur compounds protecting the liver and also enhancing its function of hormonal balance and toxin elimination.

Walnuts: remember we said that for a good plant-based diet, nuts should be your best friend. Walnuts are such a kind since they cleanse the liver of ammonia and are a good source of fiber and fatty acids.

Grapefruit: rich in antioxidants and vitamin c, these help the liver burn fat through the compound known as naringenin, and also aid detoxification.

Lemon: Whether you add lemon to your drink, foods, as juice, or simply squeezing it in warm water, you are doing a fine job acquiring proper digestion, boosting the production of bile in the liver, and optimizing bowel movement. Lemon is better taken in the morning or before dinner.

Milk Thistle: this is a great herb that addresses issues such as yeast infection, toxicity, hepatitis, eczema, tissue and organ healing, as well as cholesterol management in the body. You can either blend it or dissolve it in your tea.

Berries: rich in antioxidants, berries are a great help in detoxification.

Would you like even more foods on display? Then take a look at this:

DETOXIFYING VEGETABLES		
Leafy Greens	Starchy Veggies	Cruciferous
Radicchio	Winter roots like parsnips, turnips, and beets	Broccoflower
Cilantro		Broccoli
Dandelion		Broccoli sprouts
Spinach		Kale
Parsley		Cauliflower
		Cabbage
		Radishes
		Kohlrabi
		Turnips
		Collards
		Mustard
		Spinach
		Watercress

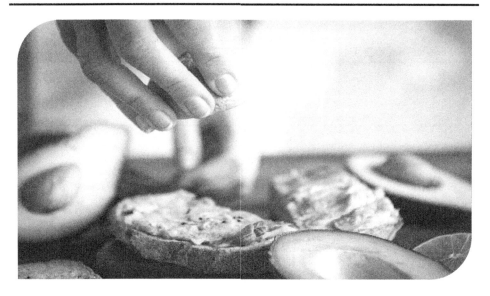

DETOXIFYING FRUITS, NUTS, SEEDS AND GRAINS

Fruits	Grains	Nuts and seeds
Blackberries	Buckwheat	Almonds
Blueberries	Brown rice	Brazil nuts
Cherries	Millet	Coconut (unsweetened)
Grapes	Quinoa	Flax seed (ground)
Papaya	Sorghum	Hazelnuts
Pineapple	Teff	pecans
Pomegranate	Whole wheat	Pine nuts
Raspberries		Pumpkin seeds
Strawberries		Sunflower
		Seed kernels

AMINO ACIDS

Meat	Legumes	Poultry	Fish
Buffalo	Peas	Turkey	Sardines
Lamb	Beans	Skinless chicken	
venison	Lentils		

FATS AND OIL

Coconut virgin oil

Flax seed (cold and pressed)

Grape seed

Extra virgin olive oil

Now, check out these detoxifying recipes.

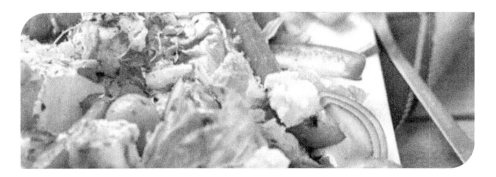

No Mozza Cheese Classic Caprese Salad

<u>Ingredients</u>

- 1 large tomato
- ½ cup of tofu, extra firm and cut in cubes
- 1 tablespoon of balsamic vinegar
- Fresh large basil leaves
- Sea salt
- Cracked pepper
- 3 garlic cloves, chopped or minced
- Olive oil

<u>How To:</u>

1. Pour a little balsamic vinegar in a small serving dish
2. Slice the tomato into ¼ inch thick rounds
3. Slice the block of tofu and slice it as thinly as the tomato
4. Add salt and pepper, and lay a basil leaf on top. Drizzle olive oil on it afterwards
5. Place a slice of tofu on the basil leaf
6. Drizzle balsamic ginger on it. Then add salt, pepper and a pinch of garlic
7. Add another tomato layer on top and repeat the pattern
8. Serve and enjoy!

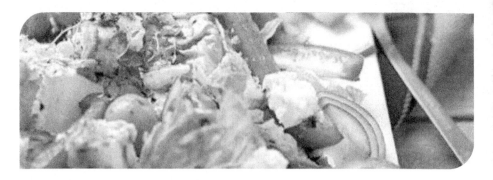

Yummy Ginger Stir-Fry

<u>Ingredients</u>

- 1½ cloves of garlic, crushed
- 2 teaspoons of chopped fresh ginger root, split
- 2 tablespoons of olive oil
- 1 small head of broccoli, cut into florets
- ½ cup of snow peas
- ¾ cup of julienned carrots
- ½ cup of sprouts
- 1 tablespoon of sea salt
- 2½ tablespoons of water
- ¼ cup of chopped onion

<u>How To:</u>

1. In a large bowl, blend garlic, 1 teaspoon of ginger and sea salt
2. Mix in broccoli, snow pea, sprouts, green beans and carrots.
3. Toss to lightly coat
4. Stir in water
5. Mix in onion, remaining one teaspoon of ginger
6. Cook until vegetables are tender but crisp
7. Serve and enjoy!

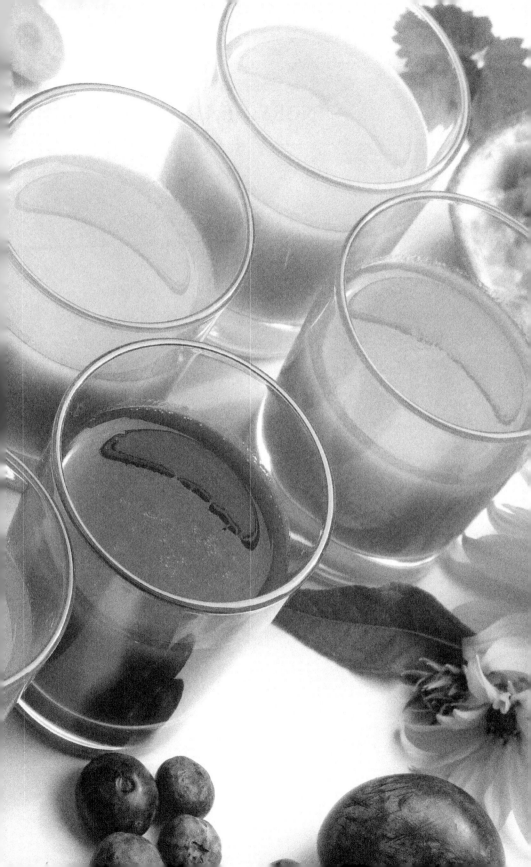

INGREDIENTS

Ginger Lemonade	Green Reboot
1 bunch of wheatgrass	4 Swiss chard leaves
1 lemon	2 apples
4 apples	1 cucumber
2 carrots	½ lemon
1 piece of ginger	1 piece of ginger
Green Tea	**Fruity splash**
1 cup of water	½ cup of almond milk
1 tablespoon of flaxseed	4 celery stalks
1 cup of raspberries	1 cucumber
1 banana	1 cup of kale
¼ cup of spinach	½ of a green apple
1 tablespoon of almond butter	½ a lime, squeezed
2 teaspoons of lemon juice	1 tablespoon of melted coconut oil
	1 cup of pineapple
Detox juice	**Simple kids' juice**
½ cups of coconut water	4 apples
1 cup of blueberries	1 carrot
½ a cup of mango	1 handful of spinach
1 cup of kale	
1 tablespoon of lemon juice	**OR**
¼ avocado	1 small beet
¼ teaspoon of cayenne pepper	2 carrots
1 tablespoon of flaxseed	2 apples
	1 handful of kale

CHAPTER 5

The Real Deal With Keto, Inflammation, Cholesterol & Diabetes

Ketogenic diet has consistently blazed the trail over the years as an effective method of nipping inflammation in the bud, managing cholesterol, and controlling diabetes. It is then no wonder why it presents a huge base of fans and followers. This being said, it is important to note that ketogenic diets function in this way to boldly cut down the level of sugar in the body (thanks to the slashing of carbs in diets. Remember we said earlier that one of the end products of carbohydrate is sugar) and gluten. The absence of this, coupled with the presence of high fat and moderate protein help to take down inflammation in battle, and also in the process of tackling diabetes and cholesterol simultaneously. Now, is that not something admirable about being on a ketogenic diet, especially a plant-based one? Speaking of inflammation, cholesterol, and diabetes, I am pretty sure a lot of us have heard one or two things about them but absolutely want to know more. Well, this is why this book is here for you, serving as a guide into the deep and cloudy mysteries of nature, particularly the overall wholeness of self-existence. So, why not come along as we dish out facts, figures, myths, and practical remedies in great detail. Get ready for the ride of your life...

All About Inflammation

It is quite a well-known fact by now, that foreign bodies get into our bodies at one point or the other. In the body, there are some cells that are naturally designed to have our backs, serving as a form of authentication, authorization, and security check against these foreign bodies.

They seem to scream to them, "What are you doing in this territory, can you show us your identification card?". Funny thing is that these toxic and/or foreign bodies always have a façade of legitimate business in the body. Now, if the soldier cells are properly taken care of, fully armed to the teeth, you can be sure they would defend you with all they have got.

If you were able to catch on with the little scenario I was trying to paint, then you can understand that there are cells in the body, the soldier cells known as the white blood cells. They differ completely from the red blood cells which produce blood, the bright red fluid in the body (the blood actually gets this red color due to the presence of a coloring agent inherent in the cells, known as hemoglobin) and serves as the very life of any human on earth. On the other hand, the white blood cells are substances produced by the body to ward off infections, viruses, and bacteria which are potential risks to the health of a person, in the sense that they may trigger sickness and diseases. Also, the absence of these white blood cells may trigger a breakdown of the body's defense mechanism, otherwise known as the immune system. Hence, the body becomes vulnerable to all forms of attack.

Inflammation may be seen as the body's biological (natural) response to irritation in a bid to let you be aware of the presence of something unusual so you can take necessary precautions. This is very automatic, just as we yelp in pain when we get pricked by a needle or thorn, or better still, a response to stimuli. When we get an irritation of the skin or whatever part of the body, we begin to feel extremely uneasy or uncomfortable. Then, we may begin to scratch all over or notice swellings or redness. While some inflammations can be slight, others may be critical enough to show the beginnings of much more severe illnesses or diseases such as cancer and rheumatoid arthritis. Where inflammations are found to be severe, they may be caused either by arteries that become enlarged as a result of so much more blood flows to the affected area, or caused by what is known as neutrophils, white blood cells filled with little sacs of enzymes and digest microorganisms. Hence, it is noticed that the condition does not get better after a few days, and may in fact extend to weeks, months, or even years. On the other hand, some inflammations may actually just be ordinary. All the same, it is better to be safe than sorry. So, how would you know if any part of your body is experiencing an inflammation?

1. The inflamed portion may turn red. This is not such a nice sight to behold, especially when you are fair-skinned or the inflamed part is visible to other people, such as having one on your nose. Now, you experience that redness because there are some finely connected tubelike structures in the body known as the capillaries. They form a well-structured network necessary for blood circulation, but when much more blood passes through them than normal, you experience redness in that spot.

2. You may also feel a kind of numbness in the inflamed area of your body, coupled with the inability to move that part comfortably

3. In consonance with numbness of the inflamed part of the body is pain. I am sure everyone must have experienced a painful or touchy part at one point or the other, so you are familiar with the sharp pain that makes you gasp "ouch" out loud, depending on the severity of the pain. Basically, pain occurs when the nerve endings of the affected area become so sensitive even to the slightest form of touch or pressure.

4. Swelling may also be the effect of an inflammation. This may also be an abscess, that is a cavity caused by tissue destruction, usually because of infection, filled with pus and surrounded by inflamed tissue

5. With pain and redness comes heat. Hence, heat is a naturally warm effect of inflammation.

At this point, I would like to stress the fact that these five symptoms of inflammation are specifically related to inflammation of the skin. However, internal organs also experience irritations and all. Examples of this are lung inflammation, flu, severe appendicitis, dermatitis, bronchitis, asthma, tuberculosis, periodontitis, hepatitis, peptic ulcer, and so on. In addition to this, in the case of severe inflammation, some of the symptoms include:

1. **Chest pain:** in case you are feeling a kind of constriction in your chest, you might just be having some reactions to foreign bodies.
2. **Abdominal pain:** pain is pain, be it in the chest, abdomen, or any part of the body. Essentially, any sensitive point in your body needs fast attention, as chronic inflammation is more often than not, associated with abdominal pain.
3. **Joint pain:** joints are points where two or more bones meet. They help us to move certain parts of our bodies. So, you will find a joint in your ankle, elbow, shoulder, and so on. The moment you begin to have acute and sensitive pain, know that a chronic illness might be setting in. Besides, you will realize that you are unable to move the joints freely.
4. **Rash:** this is something you notice as a sprinkling of not-so-good-looking dots on your skin. In fact, they may be a widely dispersed rash or more populated on the affected part of the skin. Rash is a pointer to the fact that something may be potentially going wrong. So, it would be advisable to take the necessary precautions.
5. **Mouth sores:** one thing you should never be caught having is a mouth sore. One, it severely hampers your talking and eating. Above all, it puts you in extreme pain and difficulty. But so you know, it is also a symptom of inflammation
6. **Fever:** have you ever had your temperature running at an all-time high and chills running down your body at the same time? Fever is its name. It is the culprit of this great discomfort, a potential symptom of inflammation.
7. **Fatigue:** this is the extreme sense of tiredness you feel. Inflammation says you will be continually tired if not nipped in the bud.

Having considered the cause, symptoms, and effects of inflammation, the question remains, "can it be avoided or cured?" The answer to this question is, "absolutely! There are solutions." Check these out:

- **Medications:** these are basically prescriptions doctors give you after you have been diagnosed with an illness caused by some factors, one of which is inflammation. Medications such as glucocorticoids are prescribed to treat illnesses such as inflammatory bowel disease, dermatitis, asthma, hepatitis, allergies, and arthritis, while creams, eyedrops, or ointments are given for inflammations of the eyes, nose, skin, and bowels. Other medications may include mineralocorticoids for hormonal balance and so on. However, they have been discovered to cause certain side effects such as high blood pressure, weakness of the connective tissues, low potassium levels, and so on.

- **Herbal supplements:** while it is always advisable to go to a doctor for authorization of herbal supplements and their compatibility with your health. Herbs have been found to be an alternative medical treatment. An example of a good herb is the grapple plant, otherwise known as the wood spider or devil's claw, and it is similar to sesame plants. Studies have been carried out to reveal their effective components, especially with the ability to be anti-inflammatory.

Ginger also serves as a herbal supplement that has been used for years unending and has been found to be similarly effective in its function of treating illnesses such as gastrointestinal issues, constipation, acne, dyspepsia, arthritis, and so on. Today, it is commonly used in the household to spice food, while it is greatly recommended for a great ketogenic diet.

Turmeric is another herbal supplement used worldwide as a spice, apart from its researched usefulness in curing inflammation, arthritis, and Alzheimer's disease, thanks to an active ingredient found in it: curcuma. It is also a great spice for any ketogenic diet.

Hyssop is also a herb effective especially when combined with other herbs. It is widely used in treating lung inflammation and convulsion.

At this point, I would like to add a fun fact to herbal medications, and this is the use of cannabis. Did you know that cannabis is a very good herb shown to have played active roles in treating inflammation? However, this plant has been exploited for opioid use which makes it illegal in many countries of the world today.

Keto And Inflammation

Do you remember that at one point in this book, we mentioned the fact that ketogenic foods, especially plant-based ones, must be essentially rich in fats, moderate in proteins, and really low in carbs? Well, here it is. Nuts such as walnuts and almonds, olive oil, leafy green veggies like kale and spinach, tomatoes, fatty fish such as salmon and mackerel, and so on have been discussed as forming great plant-based keto diets. In light of this, these foods, oils, and veggies are essential in playing the role of reducing inflammation and the risk of being its victim. On the other hand, foods like fast foods, fried foods, red meat, sugars that may be obtained from soda or concentrated drinks and canned drinks, pastries, and so much more are to be avoided, not just because plant-based ketogenic diets prescribe that for healthy living but also because they support the exposure of your immune system to degradation, leading to the invitation of inflammation into the body system.

Getting Rid Of Diabetes

According to the World Health Organization, diabetes is an illness that is of global prevalence. As a matter of fact, studies show that it is even more widely spread among low-income countries. In 2016, most deaths that were recorded were traced down to diabetes, estimated at about 1.6 million while people who lived up to 70 years and died had their deaths traced to a large amount of glucose and sugar in the blood. Now, how does diabetes pop up?

Diabetes, like most illnesses, does not just pop up in a day but is the consequence of a gradual process. Essentially, there is an organ in the body known as the pancreas, located just behind the stomach. This is important for the production of insulin, a hormone that plays the role of regulating the amount of sugar in the blood. Hence, when the function of the pancreas is hampered, blood sugar might spike, resulting in hyperglycemia and other diseases such as stroke and heart disease.

Upon regular checkups, doctors should tell you that your blood sugar must not exceed the level of 126 milligrams per deciliter (mg/dL). But then, there is also a condition known as "Pre-diabetes". This is otherwise known as borderline diabetes. If the level of sugar in the blood ranges from

100 to 125 milligrams per deciliter (mg/dL), then you should be careful. It means your blood sugar level is high, only that it is not high enough to constitute diabetes outright. Symptoms of pre-diabetes are similar to the Type 2 kind of diabetes. These include high blood pressure, gestational diabetes, being overweight, and having a high-density lipoprotein cholesterol level that is lower than 40 to 50 milligrams per deciliter (mg/dL).

Causes of diabetes may range from situations where either the pancreas is unable to produce any insulin, where it produces too little, or even where no response is gotten from the body cells to insulin production. So you see, it is quite a serious illness. I find it very essential, at this point to do a little breakdown of the digestive system, especially in relation to insulin production.

Quite alright, you know that zillions of cells are biologically present in your body performing various simple or complex roles. When food is taken into the body, it goes through a process of breaking down into simpler forms, one of which process is to break down into a form of sugar known as glucose. Glucose is what the body uses in energy production and it is circulated in the bloodstream. Insulin, therefore, comes into action at this point, making sure that just the right quantity of glucose is circulated around the body. I am sure you know that too much or too little of essential hormones in the body is bad and risky. The liver also supports the pancreas in energy production, serving as the storehouse of excess energy. So when the body has a low sugar level in the blood (hypoglycemia), the liver swings into action.

Diabetes is a disease that, once present, is there to stay for an entire lifetime of a person. It is worthy to note the data collected by the American Diabetes Association, stating that diabetes is the seventh leading cause of death in the United States of America., and complications such as stroke, kidney disease, heart disease, ulcers, foot disease, blindness, numbness, diabetic neuropathy, yeast infections, erectile dysfunction, tingling of the hands and feet, genital irritations and itching, slow healing wounds or cuts, and so much more may result therefrom. Although no cure has been found for it, proper management is the only option open to people living with it. In the long run, if nothing is done to control diabetes, other organs of the body are affected. It is worth taking into consideration, the fact that over 30% of the total population of people living in the United States of America, who are 18 years and above, have been diagnosed with diabetes.

Depending on the type of diagnosis, diabetes can be managed effectively, and proper management can improve the lives of people living with it. So, here go the types of diabetes:

1. **Type I diabetes:** this is the type of diabetic illness that happens when the body cannot produce insulin at all. This may be the result of destroyed cells of the pancreas, otherwise known as the beta cells, by the immune system. It is mostly found in people who are relatively young, say about 20 years of age. Type I diabetes is also known as juvenile diabetes or insulin-dependent diabetes. Symptoms of this type of diabetes, therefore, include higher degrees of thirst, incessant urination, weight loss, blurry vision, hunger pangs, and weariness.

2. **Type 2 diabetes:** otherwise known as non-insulin dependent diabetes, it originates from the body's inability to effectively process insulin, thereby resulting in a person being overweight or having excess physical activities. This essentially produces a marked difference to the Type I diabetes status, in that the body produces insulin but it is either just not enough secretion or the cells in the body do not recognize insulin for what it is and what it should be used for. Studies have shown that a larger percentage of the global population has this type of diabetes, children inclusive. The estimated number of people living with Type 2 diabetes in the United States record as high as 18 million. It is even more evident in overweight persons, people who have lived for over 40 years, and may get even worse by leading to complications such as blindness, chronic kidney failure requiring dialysis, amputations, and so on.

3. **Gestational diabetes:** from the word "gestational", it is quite easy to guess what type of diabetes this is. Sometimes during pregnancy, hormones in the body may fluctuate, thanks to estrogens and progesterone, the reproductive and pregnancy hormones but after childbirth (approximately six weeks thereafter) glucose levels in the blood are usually balanced. During pregnancy, the body is usually not as sensitive to insulin as usual, and these hormones may greatly

affect the rate at which insulin is secreted by the pancreas. Gestational diabetes is found in about 4% of all pregnancies. If gestational diabetes is discovered during screening, immediate action should be taken. It may actually be traced to family history or occurring in pregnant women who have lived for over 25 years of age.

Managing Diabetes

Diabetes can be managed quite effectively, although no cure has been found for it yet. In 2018, doctors were permitted to prescribe some medications to people with some chronic kinds of illnesses. These include:

1. **SLGT2 inhibitors:** This is a new type of medication that helps in ebbing the level of glucose in the blood. However, users have been discovered to be prone to urinary and genital infections.

2. **Metformin:** This is a medication prescribed for those who have Type 2 diabetes. It may be given in pill or liquid form and functions in lowering blood sugar, while also making insulin in the body more effective. Weight loss has also been attributed to the use of metformin. This has a huge impact on curbing diabetes

3. **Self-monitoring:** this, more than anything is a great method of managing diabetes, as self-check is safer than presumptions. This is also because the person living with diabetes has much more roles to play in ensuring that he is doing the right thing to maintain his health, the appropriate time to use his medications, making sure he takes in the proper diet, and engages in regular exercises. Self-monitoring should be done at periodic intervals, while also checking with a physician just to be on the safe side. There is a machine that enhances this self-monitoring method of managing diabetes; it is known as the self-monitoring blood glucose (SMBG) machine. This machine has a meter, lancet, and test strip that prick the skin to collect a small quantity of blood. How do you use this machine:

   • Ensure your hands are clean and dry before touching the test strips or meter. It is even more important to clean the point from which you want to draw blood with soap and warm water. This is to avoid food particles and germs from altering the readings of the machine

- If you are terrified by the process of having to prick yourself to draw blood, choosing a small and thin lancet may be the best choice for your comfort.
- Carefully take blood from the side of either your middle finger, ring finger, or little finger. Doing this won't make you feel much pain.
- Rather than putting pressure on the site from which blood would be drawn, it is better to tease blood out
- Dispose of the lancet immediately after use
- Carefully avoid exposing the meter and test strip to moisture. This is to prevent an alteration of readings, while it is also advisable not to use it more than once.
- Always check the expiry date of the machine, while it is also essential for you to close the canisters immediately after use
- Keep the machine in a cool, dry place at all times
- There may be a code requirement for older meters before use. So you might have to ensure that whatever self-monitoring machine you are using requires a code or not
- Ensure that you take the self-monitoring machine to a health care centre or a doctor to double-check its effectiveness.

Along with the self-monitoring machine is the glucometer, a portable machine for checking the glucose level in the blood. Essentially, people living with Type 1 diabetes can make use of this glucometer to know the number of insulin shots they need.

4. **Maintaining a healthy diet:** being diagnosed with diabetes does not mean the end of the world. It is never an avenue to be depressed, as this has caused more people to die before their actual deaths. More often than not, physicians prescribe a dietary change for diabetic patients or even refer him or her to a nutritionist for proper counseling. This change of dietary lifestyle plays a great role in giving a diabetic patient a quality lifespan. This being said, we will now take a look at the nutritional changes necessary to be made.

- Fresh foods are highly nutritional. Eating foods like whole grains, vegetables, proteins, and fruits will go a long way in maintaining your digestive system and metabolism. Nuts are also good for the health of anyone living with diabetes. Whole grains have been found to reduce the risk of diabetes because it really maintains the sugar level in the blood. Eating plenty of foods that have fiber content has also been highly recommended since they also reduce the risk of diabetes and heart disease and also help you lose weight. So if you have been eating concentrated foods, processed foods with additives, it is high time you stopped!

- Alcohol consumption should be reduced if you are taking it in excess. This is because alcohol thrusts more burdens on the kidneys and liver in detoxification, or better still, body cleansing. Pregnant women are sternly warned against excess alcohol and smoking. This is because it also has a direct impact on the fetus and may cognitively or physically have them impaired when they are born. Besides, diabetes may be inherited.

- Exclude, if possible, foods that have much sugars or foods that are high in calories. These include sodas, fried foods, and any other foods that have additives. This being said, it is important to bring to bear that foods high in carbs automatically mean your body extracts sugars from them, and this is not good for you. This is why a plant-based ketogenic diet ensures that your diets have just the right composition of nutrients – low carbs, moderate protein, and high fats.

- Check your body mass index (BMI) regularly, especially if you have a Type 2 diabetic case. Having a body mass index of 30 or over 30 puts you at risk of high cholesterol, which also is bad for you as a diabetic patient.

- You should also check your blood pressure regularly; ensure it does not go beyond 130/80

- Also, check your cholesterol and lipid (triglyceride) levels constantly

Having said this, it is not difficult to relate the importance of ketogenic diets, especially plant-based ketogenic diets, since it requires that you eat fresh foods, whole grains, nuts, and vegetables. A ketogenic diet also advocates for no sugar, no additives, no sweeteners, no processed foods, reduced alcohol, and low carbs, keeping your blood glucose close to normal by balancing your diet with medications, as prescribed by your health care provider.

Cholesterol

Cholesterol is a kind of waxy and fatty substance found in the blood. It is very helpful in the right quantity. For instance, it helps to build good and strong cell walls, food digestion, hormonal production, and vitamin D production. While it is a good thing to have cholesterol in the body, too much of it is dangerous to your health, especially the heart. This happens when triglycerides, a kind of fat present in the blood, has a high percentage, thereby making a person prone to heart disease.

There are essentially two types of cholesterol:

1. Low-density lipoproteins (LDL)
2. High-density lipoproteins (HDL)

Low-density lipoproteins are otherwise known as the bad type of cholesterol because it circulates cholesterol round the body, and hardens the walls of the arteries of the heart, narrowing and hardening them. This leads to a complication known as atherosclerosis which can also reduce the amount of blood flowing through the arteries.

Measurements of low-density lipoproteins cholesterol level should normally be less than 100 milligrams per deciliter (mg/dL). Hence, when it shoots as high as 190 milligrams per deciliter (mg/dL), know that you are already in the danger zone. On the other hand, High-density lipoproteins are a good type of lipoproteins that help to transport excess cholesterol to the liver. Therefore, readings of HDL levels should be 60 milligrams per deciliter (mg/dL) or even higher.

Causes Of High Cholesterol

High cholesterol may be traced to a number of factors. One of these is eating saturated fats and trans fats present in foods such as deep-fried foods, processed foods, chocolates, dairy products, animal foods, meat, and so on. Research has shown that high cholesterol may actually be genetic. This means if you have a family history of high cholesterol, just like a family history of diabetes, you are at the risk of having one too. This genetic condition is known as inherited familial hypercholesterolemia, with shooting LDL levels. Hence, there is a need to put checks on it.

Poor diets are a one-way ticket to increasing cholesterol levels in the blood, especially when they are all made up of saturated fats found in some commercially baked foods, crackers, and microwave popcorns. Red meat and full-fat dairy products which increase cholesterol levels should also be avoided. Always have it at the back of your mind that plant-based keto diets do the trick more often than not, and they are by far better than animal-based diets, which makes you vulnerable to all sorts of illnesses and diseases.

Many people do not also pay attention to their weight. Eating just about anything is a gross habit that should stop immediately. As we have stated before, over thirty percent (30%) of people living in the United States of America are living with Diabetes, which is a direct cause of high cholesterol levels in the blood. Hence, obesity places a person at a greater risk of high cholesterol, diabetes, and other complications of health.

If you are the kind of person who is just too lazy for workouts or exercises, care should be taken. Exercises help to boost the body's supply of good cholesterol, otherwise known as HDL while decreasing bad cholesterol – LDL.

Alcoholism and smoking have also been discovered as risk factors for high cholesterol. This is because they potentially damage the walls of the blood vessels such as veins and arteries, making them prone to an accumulation of fatty deposits, while also contributing to lowering the level of good cholesterol (HDL) available in your body.

Other causes may be due to the presence of diabetes, the condition whereby the thyroid gland is underproductive or inefficient, the effect of female hormones like estrogens and progesterone, pregnancy, polycystic ovary syndrome, liver or kidney disease, drugs that shoot up the LDL cholesterol and decrease the HDL cholesterol, examples of which are anabolic steroids, corticosteroids, progestins, and so on.

According to a report from Harvard health, there are certain foods that actively decrease cholesterol levels. These include beans, eggplant, and okra, nuts, vegetable oil such as canola and sunflower, barley and whole grains, oats, fruits such as apples, grains, citrus, and strawberries, fishes such as salmon, sardines, and tuna, foods rich in fiber, and so on. On the contrary, then, certain foods must be avoided. These include red meat, margarine, hydrogenated oils, and so on. This being said, it is evident that these foods are highly recommended by the ketogenic nutritional diet, especially a plant-based diet at that. So, you see, cholesterol can be effectively cured by plant-based ketogenic diets.

Having a high cholesterol level in the blood often leads to:

1. Heart attack: heart attack is often caused when there is a shortage or absence of blood flow into the heart. How does this happen? Where there is a rupture or a tear in the artery, blood clots may form, thereby preventing the free passage of blood through the artery. This is what happens when a person suffers a heart attack.
2. Chest pain: depending on the severity of the problem, a person may experience chest pain due to a concentrated level of cholesterol in the blood. Otherwise known as angina, chest pain occurs when the arteries are affected by excess cholesterol. Hence, your chest hardens, and feels tight or constricted, like you need air.
3. Stroke: stroke is a consequence of heart failure. When a blood clot prevents blood flow to the brain, there arises a failure.

Is A High Cholesterol Level In The Blood Preventable?

Absolutely! Basically, if you are looking forward to having a quality lifespan, then you have to adopt a quality lifestyle. This entails quitting smoking since it contributes to hardening the walls of veins and arteries, vessels that circulate blood around the body; you also need to quit every form of alcohol too. It is safer this way since it works hand in hand with smoking in hardening the walls of veins and arteries.

It is advisable to begin a plant-based ketogenic diet since they encourage eating healthy foods, vegetables, and whole grains and sternly warn against processed foods, sugars, concentrated drinks, fried foods, and animal-based products, junks, and fast foods. Even if you do not have to transition completely to the plant-based ketogenic lifestyle, you could at least do yourself a favor by including it in your diet at least three times a week. Now that studies have shown that even children are prone to the risk of living with diabetes, your children also have to be monitored in the kind of diet they take in.

Cultivating the habit and culture of exercising your body is a good choice if you are looking towards increasing the level of good cholesterol in the body, and simultaneously decreasing the level of bad cholesterol.

Moderation in everything we do is one of the precious keys to living a healthy life. So, monitor yourself and leave out the bad habits that are unfavorable to your health. Ensure that you sleep well while also eating well. Stress is a risk factor for many forms of illnesses and diseases. Of course, they always start small and if not curbed, they escalate. Your mental health is precious and should be considered so by you too. The older you get, the more careful you should be about taking care of yourself. This is because many things start to change in the body system. For instance, the kidneys and the livers start to gradually slow down in their functions, and you may feel more easily stressed. So you have to regularly check in with your doctor, nutritionist, or any other health provider of your choice. Adults as well as children should have appointments with the doctor so that appropriate tests can be conducted, especially for persons with a genetic element or family history of high cholesterol or diabetes, high blood pressure, heart diseases, and so on.

CONCLUSION PLANT BASED KETO

Transitioning to a plant-based diet after a whole lifetime of eating meat and all other animal-based diets can be quite difficult. But if you have taken the pain to go through every page of this book, then it is my hope that I have been able to convince you about the benefits of having at least greens in your daily meals. While your body may take a while to adapt, I can assure you that the best of advantages is enjoyed by this same body. Never mind all the buzz around you, all you simply need to do is take a deep breath and take it one day at a time. Before you know it, it has become second nature to you.

Ketogenic diets, especially a plant-based one is highly beneficial in that it helps your body seek alternative form of energy known as ketones, while also helping your body get into ketosis and maintain it. If you are looking towards losing some weight or maintaining your trim body, it is good to at least include plant-based keto into your diet. Diabetic patients also have a lot to gain by eating plant-based foods, whole grains, leafy veggies and lots more. Cholesterol levels get reduced by them, and you find the most appropriate way of avoiding chronic diseases that may invade your body system and live with you for the rest of your life with plant-based diets.

Life couldn't be easier with the amazing recipes to make the whole ride fun and creative. Eating just the right amounts of carbs, fats and proteins is the ideal choice for a healthy plant-based ketogenic diet. Feel free to try out any of the above recipes or get a cookbook for more. There is really a whole wide world of experience and nutrition to gain from trying them out. If you are also looking to having your trim waist and body back, this book is also for you. Even if you cannot be a veggie freak, it would be nice to at least try it out about 3 times a week.

Let go of risks of diabetes, inflammation, heart diseases, gastro-intestinal infections, cancer and cholesterol with tasty plant-based diets.

Surely, you can never be wrong having them as snacks, smoothies and desserts. At any time of the day, you are good to go with plant-based nutritious foods. Remember, low carbs, high fat and moderate protein. Hmmm, even when I was looking everywhere for special recipes, all I could do was savor while writing.

I've got to drop my pen to try some recipes out myself. I mustn't lose out on this. So, thank you for accompanying me all through the ride. I truly hope you found it worth the while.

KETO
Vegan Cookbook

BY LARA RUSH

The ketogenic diet is a high-fat (about 75 percent of total calories), low-carb (20-40), moderate-protein diet that has been pushed for its dramatic weight loss and overall health benefits. Although this manner of eating is commonly linked with animal meals, it may be altered to meet plant-based meal patterns, including vegan diets.

Vegan diets exclude all animal products, making low-carb eating more challenging. Vegans, on the other hand, can gain the potential benefits of a ketogenic diet with proper preparation. Vegans who eat high-fat, plant-based foods like coconut oil, avocados, seeds, and almonds can achieve ketosis.

Given that both vegan and keto diets may enhance your health in comparable ways, combining the two by adopting a keto vegan diet is likely to have a very good influence on your health.

Weight loss, improved blood sugar control, lower LDL (bad) cholesterol, balanced HDL (good) cholesterol, reduced risk of obesity-related disorders, and lowered heart disease risk factors are just a few of the health advantages of Keto Vegan Recipes.

CHAPTER 6

30 Tasty Vegetarian Keto Recipes To Go

I'm so excited we finally are at the "menu menu" segment of this book. Guess I'm not the only one who's been looking forward to this. Now that you have learned so much about the theory of the plant-based ketogenic diet, this is the practical aspect of it. This chapter will show you how to be creative with your diets, so you do not feel so restricted. You also get to have your mind exposed to different combinations of food with low carbs, high fat, and moderate protein without any processed additive, just as you would get to love it to bits. Now is the time to evict every sense of deprivation or loss, because, in fact, you get to benefit more. Instead of opting for meals offered at restaurants every time, try making your foods from scratch. You will soon find out that the recipes provided here will not take too much of your time. Remember to include this in your children's diets too. As a family, there is also a lot to gain, not only for body weight loss purposes. So, it is high time you revamped your pantry and started being more interested in lemon drinks, meals, and smoothies. With this, I hope you will say an honest goodbye to fast foods, sugars, additives, and all the junks that come in beautiful packages. Share in the health benefits and nourishment of thirty amazing and exquisite dishes. Whether you take it as your breakfast, lunch, snack, dinner, or dessert, you are good to go. Well, here it is! So, let's get started...

Keto Vegan Porridge

Servings: 02

Preparation time: 5 minutes

Cook time: 2 minutes

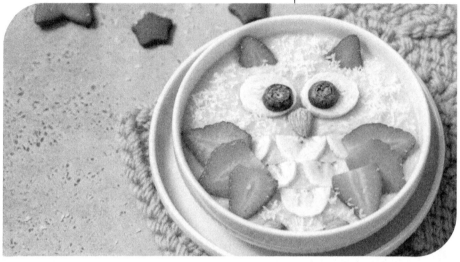

A well-balanced blend of seeds is the key to a creamy keto vegan porridge. In only a few minutes, you can cook a delicious keto vegan breakfast with this recipe.

Ingredients

- 15 g ground flaxseeds
- 220 ml full-fat coconut milk
- a pinch of cinnamon
- 1 cup unsweetened shredded coconut
- 35 g frozen blueberries
- 15 g fresh raspberries
- 35 g chia seeds
- a pinch of salt

Directions

1. Combine the seeds, spices, and full-fat coconut milk in a mixing bowl. Allow for a 10-minute rest period.

2. In a blender or food processor, combine the ingredients. Blend in a pinch of salt until the mixture is smooth.

3. Place the ingredients in a bowl and top with the toppings for a cold porridge.

4. Warm the mixture in a small saucepan and add more milk if necessary for a warm porridge; pour into a bowl and top with desired toppings.

Nutrition

Calories: 157.7 | Fat: 9.6g | Saturated Fat: 4g | Net Carbohydrates: 3.2g
Protein: 5.3g | Fiber: 7g | Sugar: 0.8g | Sodium: 48.9mg

Keto Vegan Tofu Scrambles

Servings: 06

Preparation time: 15 minutes

Cook time: 15 minutes

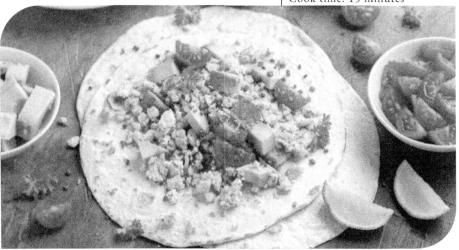

For morning scrambles, firm or extra-firm tofu is excellent since it has a compact structure that creates the right mouthfeel. This dish is a winner whether you're grabbing a meal to go before going out to work on Tuesday morning or presenting a lovely brunch on Sunday morning.

Ingredients

- 2 chopped avocado
- 5-6 kale leaves
- 5 cloves garlic (minced)
- 1 block of firm tofu (pressed)
- 1 teaspoon paprika
- 1 teaspoon ground turmeric
- ½ teaspoon sea salt
- ¼ teaspoon ground black pepper
- 1 tablespoon nutritional yeast
- ½ green onion
- 2 tablespoons almond or coconut milk
- 2 teaspoons coconut oil

Directions

1. Tofu should be pressed and sliced into pieces.

2. Cook tofu slices in coconut milk in an oiled pan over medium heat, breaking it up as it cooks.

3. To make the scramble sauce, combine nutritional yeast flakes, turmeric, paprika, and garlic powder in a mixing bowl.

4. Pour the sauce over the tofu and toss it around to coat each piece.

5. Cook until the kale and green onions are soft, about 5 minutes.

6. Add the chopped avocado and season to taste with salt and pepper.

7. Serve.

Nutrition

Calories: 157.7 | Fat: 9.6g | Saturated Fat: 4g | Net Carbohydrates: 3.2g
Protein: 5.3g | Fiber: 7g | Sugar: 0.8g | Sodium: 48.9mg

Keto Vegan Chia Seed Pudding

Servings: 02

Preparation time: 5 minutes

Cook time: 20 minutes

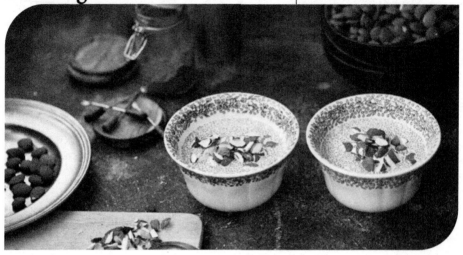

Smooth and creamy, this keto vegan chia pudding is ideal for a low-carb breakfast! It just takes 5 minutes to prepare and can be customized in a variety of ways, including vegan, whole30, and gluten-free.

Ingredients

- 170 ml unsweetened coconut milk
- 30 g strawberries (chopped into small pieces)
- 2 tsp chopped hazelnuts
- 35 g chia seeds
- 3-4 tsp chopped almonds
- 2 tsp peanut butter

Directions

1. Combine the chia seeds and coconut milk in a mixing basin.

2. Refrigerate the mixture in an airtight jar for at least 10 minutes before serving (for a better result, wait 20 minutes). You may also store the pudding in the refrigerator for up to two days.

3. Add the toppings to the chia pudding and divide it into smaller containers (strawberries, peanut butter, chopped hazelnuts, chopped almonds).

4. Serve right away.

Nutrition

Calories: 161.4 | Fat: 10.2g | Saturated Fat: 3.8g | Net Carbohydrates: 2.1g
Protein: 4.9g | Fiber: 7g | Sugar: 0.9g | Sodium: 114.5mg

Spinach Mushroom Scrambled Tofu With Vegan Cheese

Servings: 04 to 06

Preparation time: 30 minutes

Cook time: 12 minutes

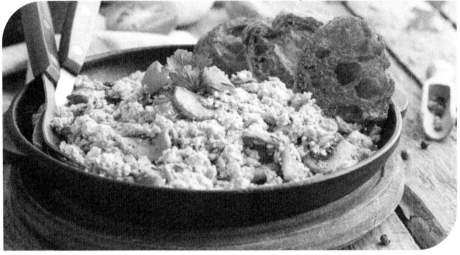

For vegans who desire an egg-like dish to start their day, a tofu scramble with spinach and mushrooms is the perfect protein boost. This tofu scramble recipe is simple to adapt to your tastes.

Ingredients

- 2 cups finely sliced mushrooms
- 1/4 tsp black pepper
- 1/2 cup vegan cheese shreds
- 1/2 cup unsweetened coconut milk
- 1 spring onions
- 14 oz block of medium-firm tofu
- 1 tsp garlic powder
- 1/4 tsp turmeric
- 1/4 tsp paprika
- 2 cups baby spinach leaves
- Salt to taste (optional)

Directions

1. Using paper towels or tea towels, pat the tofu dry. Squeeze out any extra liquid gently. Then press the tofu for at least 20 minutes in a tofu press or a heavy pan like a cast-iron skillet.

2. Crumble tofu into a large mixing dish with your hands. Crumble using the back of a fork for a finer texture.

3. Mix in all of the seasonings (excluding the salt) until everything is well blended.

4. Warm a little amount of oil over medium heat. Cook, stirring periodically, for 2 minutes after adding the tofu.

5. Pour in the coconut milk that hasn't been sweetened. If you're not sure how soft you want your scramble to be, add a tablespoon at a time until you achieve the appropriate texture.

6. Cook for 2 minutes after adding the spring onions and ginger. Cook for 4 minutes, or until the mushrooms are gently browned. Toss in the spinach

71

and allow it to wilt.

7. Stir in the vegan cheese until it has melted (about 1-2 minutes)

8. Remove from heat after the cheese has melted. If using, season with salt (use a dash at a time to avoid overpowering the tofu scramble; it's nasty stuff!)

9. You may top with chives, green onions, vegan sauce, or whatever else you like! ENJOY!

Nutrition

Calories: 203 | Fat: 13.7g | Saturated Fat: 2.1g | Net Carbohydrates: 2.6g
Protein: 15.4g | Fiber: 6.3g | Sugar: 3.1g | Sodium: 288mg

Keto Vegan Smoothie

Servings: 02

Preparation time: 4 minutes

Cook time: 0 minutes

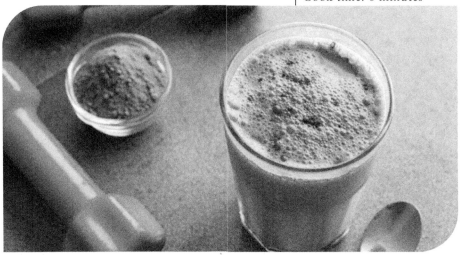

This Keto Vegan Smoothie is a great addition to your keto vegan diet. It just takes 2 minutes to prepare, has only 4 grams of net carbohydrates, and is extremely flavorful and nutritious!

Ingredients

- 1 tbsp cocoa powder
- 30 g Vegan Protein Powder chocolate
- 1 tbsp Almond or Peanut Butter
- 300 ml Full-fat coconut milk and chilled
- 1 tbsp Chia Seeds (optional)

Directions

1. In a blender, combine all of the ingredients, starting with coconut milk.
2. Blend for 30 to 45 seconds or until the mixture is smooth. Serve with strawberries on top.

Nutrition

Calories: 180.4 | Fat: 11.1g | Saturated Fat: 2.4g | Net Carbohydrates: 4g
Protein: 15.9g | Fiber: 4g | Sugar: 1g | Sodium: 209mg

Keto Vegan Tahini Halva Cake

Pieces: 08

Preparation time: 15 minutes

Chill: 2 hours

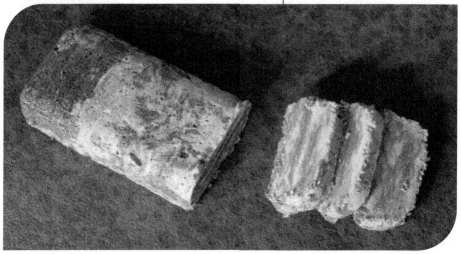

Cake for breakfast? After all, why not? This keto-friendly breakfast is a Tahini-based cake called Halva, which is popular in the Middle East and Asia. The walnuts, cacao powder, and nutty tahini give this a deliciously decadent flavor, and it's also a perfect keto vegan dessert!

Ingredients

- 3 Tbsps. cacao powder
- 1 cup Sesame tahini
- 1/2 cup walnuts
- 1 Tbsp. chia seeds
- 1 cup creamed coconut

Directions

1. To begin, coarsely grind the walnuts.
2. Then, using a hand blender, a kitchen chopper, or any other acceptable equipment, combine all of the ingredients together.
3. Fill a cake mold halfway with the mixture and chill for 2 hours to solidify.
4. Garnish with berries, desiccated coconut, hemp seeds, or any keto-friendly items you have on hand.

Nutrition

Calories: 457.8 | Fat: 38.4g | Saturated Fat: 7.6g | Net Carbohydrates: 8.1g
Protein: 10.3g | Fiber: 6.6g | Sugar: 3.1g | Sodium: 358.5mg

Keto Vegan Pancakes (Egg-Free, Dairy-Free)

Batch of Pancakes: 01

Preparation time: 5 minutes

Cook time: 10 minutes

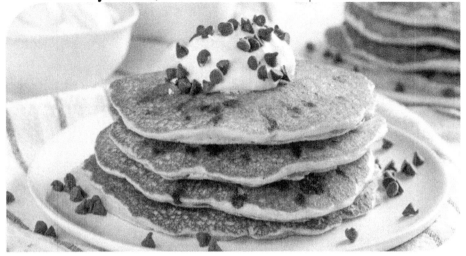

These gluten-free, low-carb vegan pancakes are ideal for a lazy weekend morning. They're devoid of dairy, eggs, soy, and sugar, and they're high in protein, fiber, and omega-3 fatty acids. The ideal and delectable pancake!

Ingredients

- 1/4 cup unsweetened almond milk
- 1 tbsp ground flax
- 1 tbsp coconut flour
- 2 tbsp unsweetened almond butter
- 1/2 tsp baking powder
- Liquid stevia or Swerve (great sweetener for diabetics) to taste
- 1 tbsp coconut oil or olive oil
- pinch of salt (if not using salted almond butter)

Directions

1. Preheat your frying pan on low, medium heat. Using your preferred oil, lightly coat the pan.

2. Combine almond butter and almond milk in a small plate.

3. Combine the dry ingredients in a separate bowl and stir until thoroughly combined.

4. Stir together the wet and dry ingredients until fully combined. Allow the flax and coconut flour to absorb the liquid for 3-5 minutes.

5. Pour the batter into your skillet and carefully spread it out to make pancakes. This yielded three 4" pancakes. Wet the back of a spoon and use it as a spatula if the batter is tough to spread.

6. Cook for 4-5 minutes, or until the pancake readily flips (check it at 3 by gently shimmying your spatula under the pancake). You want to see those small bubbles all over the surface, just like with regular pancakes.

7. Flip and cook for another 2-3 minutes until brown on the bottom.

8. Enjoy!! Top with vegan butter, coconut cream, sugar-free syrup, fruit, or additional almond butter.

Nutrition

Calories: 263.1 | Fat: 21.3g | Saturated Fat: 2.6g | Net Carbohydrates: 4.4g
Protein: 9.8g | Fiber: 8.5g | Sugar: 1.3g | Sodium: 58.7mg

Creamy Vegetable Soup

Servings: 08

Preparation time: 15 minutes

Cook time: 35 minutes

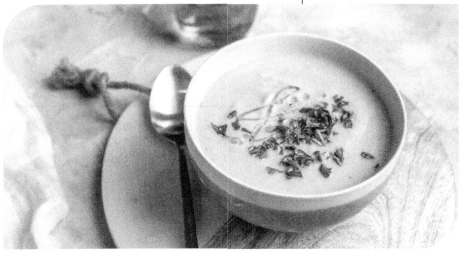

This Keto (Low-Carb) Creamy Vegetable Soup is a thick, creamy, beautifully tasty soup that may be served as a starter or as a whole meal! It's a hearty meal that you can reheat yourself or send in thermoses for your family.

Ingredients

- 1 clove garlic
- 1 small brown onion (70 g/ 2.5 oz)
- 2 celery stalks (80 g/ 2.8 oz)
- 2 tbsp butter (30 g/ 1.1 oz)
- 2 cups vegetable stock (480 ml/ 16 Fl oz)
- 2 cups water (480 ml/ 16 Fl oz)
- 1 tsp fresh thyme, plus extra for garnish
- 1/2 tsp onion powder (optional)
- 500 g zucchini (1.1 lb.)
- sea salt and pepper to

Directions

1. The veggies should be washed. Remove the cauliflower's green portions. Peel the garlic and onion.

2. In a large saucepan, melt the butter over medium to high heat. Finely chop the onion and garlic and sauté until they are translucent.

3. Combine the cauliflower, zucchini, celery, and spices in a large mixing bowl.

4. Bring the vegetable broth, along with the water, to a boil. Reduce the heat to a low and cover the pot. Cook for approximately 15 minutes or until the veggies are tender.

5. Remove from the heat and purée with an immersion mixer until smooth. Return to low heat and stir in the vegan cream until it is well cooked.

77

taste
- 1 cup vegan cream (240 ml/ 8 Fl oz)
- 700 g cauliflower (1.5 lb.)
- 4 tbsp extra virgin olive oil (60 ml)

6. Serve with a sprig of thyme and a drizzle of olive oil (approximately 1/2 tablespoon each dish).

Nutrition

Calories: 259 | Fat: 24.3g | Saturated Fat: 9.5g | Net Carbohydrates: 5.6g
Protein: 4.8g | Fiber: 2.8g | Sugar: 3.3g | Sodium: 349.6mg

Cheesy Zucchini Noodles With Walnut Pesto

Servings: 04

Preparation time: 20 minutes

Cook time: 0 minutes

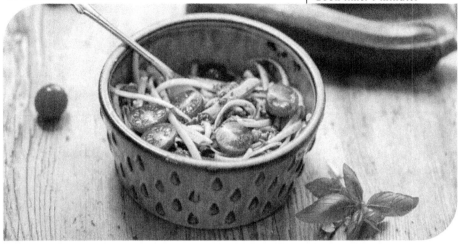

My favorite vegetarian meal, Zoodles with Walnut Pesto and Vegan Cheese, isn't complete without it throughout the summer. This is a simple, tasty, and wonderful low-carb recipe that takes only 20 minutes to prepare!

Ingredients

- 2 tbsp vegan cheese
- 4 medium dry zucchinis, spiralized and roughly chopped
- 1/4 cup lemon juice
- 2 tbsp nutritional yeast for garnish
- 2 cups parsley, roughly chopped and packed
- 2 cloves garlic, chopped
- 1/2 tsp sea salt
- 1/3 cup walnuts, soaked overnight and dehydrated at 100°F until dry, about 24 to 36 hours
- 1/4 cup olive oil

Directions

1. To make zucchini "noodles," use a spiralizer tool.

2. Combine parsley, walnuts, lemon juice, vegan cheese, garlic, and sea salt in a food processor and pulse until well blended but still chunky.

3. Slowly sprinkle in the olive oil while the machine is running, and process until fully combined. Stop as required to scrape down the bowl's sides. Continue to process until you have the consistency you want.

4. Combine zucchini noodles and pesto in a large mixing basin. Toss until the noodles are well covered, and the pesto is evenly distributed.

5. Serve with a sprinkle of nutritional yeast on top. Serve.

Nutrition

Calories: 117 | Fat: 7.6g | Saturated Fat: 0.2g | Net Carbohydrates: 4.5g
Protein: 6.4g | Fiber: 4g | Sugar: 0.1g | Sodium: 29mg

Vegetable And Tofu Soup

Servings: 04

Preparation time: 5 minutes

Cook time: 20 minutes

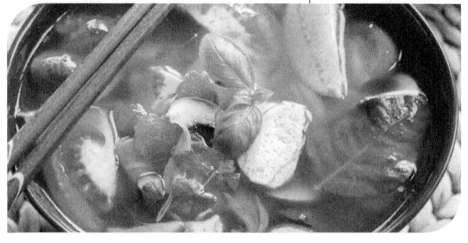

Tofu has a reputation for being bland, but in this veggie-packed keto soup, it's anything but when marinated in vegan spice for up to 2 hours. Exceptionally tasty!

Ingredients

- 2 cups reduced-sodium vegetable broth
- 2 tablespoons olive oil
- 1 (14.5 ounces) can no-salt-added diced tomatoes with basil, garlic, undrained
- 3 cups sliced fresh mushrooms (8 ounces)
- ½ cup fresh or frozen peas, thawed
- 1 pinch Shredded Vegan cheese
- 1 (12 ounces) package extra-firm, tub-style tofu (fresh bean curd), drained, and cut into 3/4-inch cubes
- ½ cup 1-inch pieces asparagus
- ½ cup chopped roasted red sweet pepper

Directions

1. In a shallow dish, place tofu in a resealable plastic bag. Combine the oil and Vegan seasoning in a mixing bowl. Close the bag and turn to coat the tofu. Refrigerate for at least 2 hours.

2. Cook over medium-high heat in a 5- to 6-quart Dutch oven coated with cooking spray. Cook, flipping once, for 5 to 7 minutes, or until tofu is golden brown.

3. Combine the veggie broth and canned tomatoes in a large mixing bowl. Bring the water to a boil. Reduce heat to low and add mushrooms, peas, and asparagus. Cook for 8 to 10 minutes, or until the veggies are barely soft. Heat through the sweet pepper, dried tomatoes, and olives.

4. Serve with vegan cheese on top if desired.

- ⅓ cup oil-packed dried tomatoes, drained and finely chopped
- 1 teaspoon dried Vegan seasoning, crushed (1 tablespoon dried oregano, 2 teaspoons dried basil, 2 teaspoons dried thyme, 1 teaspoon dried sage, ½ teaspoon dried rosemary)
- ¼ cup sliced green olives

Nutrition

Calories: 164 | Fat: 15.5g | Saturated Fat: 1.9g | Net Carbohydrates: 4.8g Protein: 16.7g | Fiber: 8.7g | Sugar: 7.1g | Sodium: 487.3mg

Creamy Coconut And Cauliflower Soup

Servings: 04

Preparation time: 15 minutes

Cook time: 45 minutes

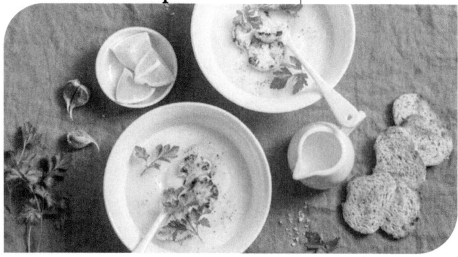

This Keto Vegan Cauliflower Soup is created with dairy-free cashew cream, roasted cauliflower, garlic, and onions and is exceptionally rich and creamy. It's gluten-free, paleo, low-carb, and Whole30 compliant, making it ideal for meal prep.

Ingredients

- 1 large cauliflower
- ¼ cup nutritional yeast
- ½ cup unsweetened almond milk
- 1 red onion
- 1.5 tbsp olive oil or avocado oil
- 4 garlic cloves
- 1 tsp mixed dried herbs
- 3 cups vegetable stock
- 2 cup cashews

Toppings (optional):

- Toasted seeds
- Finely chopped chives

Directions

1. To make the cashew cream, puree the cashews and almond milk until smooth in a high-powered blender. (If you don't have a high-powered blender, soak the cashews in boiling water for half an hour before draining them.)

2. Preheat the oven to 350 degrees Fahrenheit.

3. Place cauliflower florets on a baking pan and cut them into bite-size pieces. Coat in 1 tablespoon olive oil, salt, and pepper

4. Preheat the oven to 350°F and bake for 30-35 minutes, or until the edges begin to brown and crisp. Halfway through, give them a toss.

5. Chop the red onion finely. In a skillet/pan over medium heat, heat 1/2 tbsp oil, then add the onion and sauté for a few minutes.

6. Stir in the finely chopped garlic and dry herbs, and simmer for a few more minutes.

7. Combine the vegetable stock and roasted

cauliflower in a large mixing bowl. Simmer for 5 minutes at a low temperature.

8. Stir in the cashew cream and nutritional yeast.

9. Blend until smooth; add additional water if necessary to thin it down. Season with salt and pepper to taste.

10. Top with chopped chives and toasted seeds if desired. (Optional)

Nutrition

Calories: 212 | Fat: 13.4g | Saturated Fat: 2.6g | Net Carbohydrates: 5.1g
Protein: 8.1g | Fiber: 5g | Sugar: 1.7g | Sodium: 150mg

Keto Vegan Sesame Ginger Coleslaw

Servings: 12

Preparation time: 30 minutes

Chill: 60 minutes

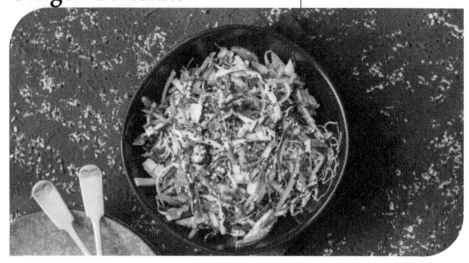

Shredded cabbage, carrots, cilantro, and green onions are mixed in an oil-free sesame ginger dressing in this keto vegan coleslaw. It's quick and easy to make, and it's full of vibrant, zesty tastes! This wonderful recipe adds texture, color, and levels of taste to any meal.

Ingredients

Sesame Ginger Dressing:

- 1 tbsp tahini
- 1 tbsp maple syrup
- 2 tbsp rice vinegar
- 2 tbsp almond butter
- 3 tbsp lime juice
- 1 tbsp hot sauce
- 1 medium garlic clove peeled
- 2 tbsp low-sodium tamari
- 2-inch knob fresh ginger peeled

Coleslaw:

- 2 cups carrots thinly sliced
- 1 cup cilantro roughly

Directions

1. In a small blender cup, combine almond butter, tahini, tamari, rice vinegar, lime juice, spicy sauce, maple syrup, garlic clove, and ginger. Blend on high until smooth and creamy.

2. In a large mixing bowl, combine the thinly sliced red and green cabbage, carrots, green onions, and cilantro. Toss the cabbage mixture with the dressing to incorporate.

3. Cover and refrigerate the coleslaw for at least an hour before serving.

chopped (add more to
taste)
- 5 cups green cabbage
thinly sliced
- 1 cup green onions
sliced
- 5 cups red cabbage
thinly sliced

Nutrition

Calories: 68.4 | Fat: 4.1g | Saturated Fat: 0.4g | Net Carbohydrates: 3.3g
Protein: 3.5g | Fiber: 3g | Sugar: 3.7g | Sodium: 217mg

Large Green Salad With Tempeh Tahini Mint Dressing

Servings: 02

Preparation time: 10 minutes

Cook time: 20 minutes

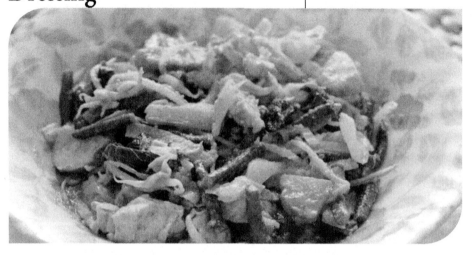

Easy and refreshing tempeh salad with ginger, garlic, spinach, and kale, plus a dash of lime juice for extra zing. In 30 minutes, you can have a nutritious, protein-rich salad!

Ingredients

- 1 large onion, finely diced
- 1 carrot, peeled and chopped
- 2 cloves of garlic, minced
- 1 shallot, minced
- 1 green onion, thinly sliced
- 1 tablespoon plant-based oil
- 1-inch fresh ginger, grated
- ½ red bell pepper, diced
- 15 ounces tempeh, finely diced
- 1 tbsp maple syrup
- ¼ tsp ground

Directions

1. Wash the mint leaves and combine them with the rest of the ingredients for the Tahini dressing in a food processor. Blend until completely smooth.

2. In a large skillet, heat the oil over medium heat. Add the onion, garlic, shallot, and ginger once the pan is heated. Cook, stirring periodically, for 5-7 minutes, or until onions are tender.

3. Red bell pepper, carrots, and tempeh chopped. Cook, occasionally stirring, for 7-8 minutes, or until carrots are cooked. To maintain some crunch, you can slightly undercook the veggies.

4. Combine the soy sauce, maple syrup, and ground coriander in a mixing bowl. Cook for another 3 to 5 minutes. Taste and adjust spices as necessary, adding extra soy sauce for saltiness and/or sriracha

coriander

- 3 tbsp soy sauce
- 2 cups chopped greens (kale, spinach, etc.)
- juice from 1 lime (or lemon)
- optional toppings: red pepper flakes, sesame seeds

Tahini Mint Dressing:

- 3 tablespoons Tahini
- 2 teaspoons Olive Oil
- 1 teaspoon Maple Syrup or 1/2 teaspoon Agave
- 4 tablespoons Water
- 3/4 teaspoon salt
- 8 fresh Mint Leaves
- 2 small Garlic Cloves
- 1/4 small Red Onion
- 1 teaspoon Paprika
- 3 tablespoons Lemon Juice

for heat, if desired.

5. Remove from the heat and toss in the chopped green onions, kale, spinach, and lime juice in a large serving dish. Allow it to cool completely before serving with Tahini Mint Dressing.

Nutrition

Calories: 373.8 | Fat: 16.7g | Saturated Fat: 4.6g | Sodium: 338mg
Net Carbohydrates: 11.4g | Protein: 28.3g | Fiber: 3.9g | Sugar: 7.8g

Cauliflower Tacos With Avocado Lime Crema

Servings: 08

Preparation time: 8 minutes

Cook time: 22 minutes

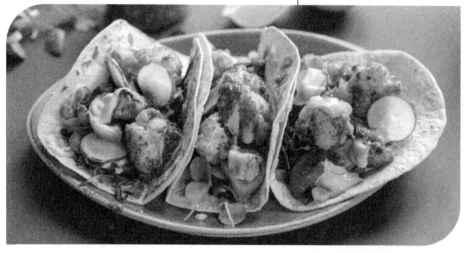

With air-fried, grilled, or roasted cauliflower, cabbage, and jalapeno drizzled with an avocado-lime crème, these Cauliflower Tacos are simple to prepare. They're gluten-free, paleo, vegan, grain-free, and low-carb, making them ideal for a light lunch! To make them Whole30 compliant, serve them in a bowl or over jicama, coconut, or lettuce wraps.

Ingredients

For the Roasted Cauliflower:

- 1 teaspoon ground cumin
- 1/4 teaspoon garlic powder
- 1 teaspoon sea salt
- 2 teaspoons chili powder
- 1 small head cauliflower (about 4 cups), washed and cut into bite-size florets
- 1 Tablespoon fresh lime juice
- 1 Tablespoon olive oil
- 1/2 teaspoon smoked paprika

Directions

To Roast the Cauliflower:

1. Preheat the oven or air fryer to 400 degrees Fahrenheit. Combine chili powder, cumin, paprika, garlic powder, and salt in a medium mixing bowl.

2. **For the oven, prepare the following:** A baking sheet should be lined or greased. Drizzle olive oil, lime, and salt over the cauliflower on the baking sheet. In a single layer, spread everything out evenly. Roast for 20-22 minutes until cauliflower is golden and soft, turning periodically. Remove the dish from the oven and set it aside.

3. **For the air fryer:** Preheat the air fryer to 400 degrees Fahrenheit. Place in the basket of an air fryer (you will need to cook them in batches). Air fry for 8-10 minutes.

For the Avocado Cream:

- 1/4 cup fresh cilantro
- 1/2 teaspoon sea salt
- 1 large ripe avocado (or 2 medium)
- juice from 1 lime, about 2 tablespoons
- 1 clove garlic

For Serving:

- 2 jalapeno slices
- 1 1/2 cups shredded lettuce and shredded cabbage, sub with coleslaw mix for easier prep
- 1 avocado, sliced
- pickled onions
- 8-12 grain-free tortillas, Cauliflower thins work well for keto. For Whole30, serve in bowls or use jicama wraps, lettuce wraps, or coconut wraps
- fresh cilantro leaves
- Lime wedges

4. **For the grill:** Preheat the grill to 375°F on medium-high. On the grill, place a grill basket or a wide piece of foil. Grill for 8-10 minutes until the cauliflower is soft and crisp.

To Make the Avocado Cream:

5. In a food processor, combine the avocado, cilantro, lime, garlic, and salt while the cauliflower roasts. Blend until completely smooth.

To Assemble the Tacos:

6. **Char the tortillas:** Heat the tortillas in a skillet over medium-high heat for 10-20 seconds OR on the grill for 2 minutes each side, with the grill open the entire time, OR directly on a gas burner for 5 seconds on each side.

7. **Assemble the tacos:** Warm tortillas with the roasted cauliflower within. Top with shredded cabbage, jalapeno, avocado, cilantro, pickled onions, and a generous drizzle of avocado sauce, as well as a squeeze of lime juice!

Nutrition

Calories: 114.5 | Fat: 8.7g | Saturated Fat: 1.4g | Net Carbohydrates: 6.6g
Protein: 7.8g | Fiber: 4.1g | Sugar: 1.9g | Sodium: 243mg

Keto Vegan Empanadas

Servings: 04

Preparation time: 20 minutes

Cook time: 20 minutes

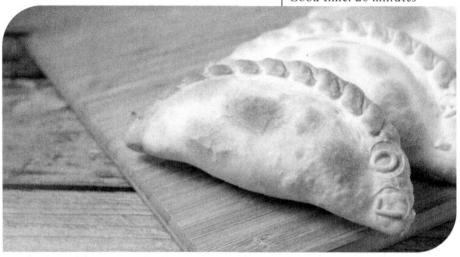

This low-carb vegan empanada dish is really easy to prepare and delicious! Crispy borders, flaky, buttery dough, and a rich filling make these rolls stand out.

Ingredients

- 1/2 cup coconut flour
- 1 teaspoon soy sauce
- 2 tablespoons psyllium husk
- 1 pinch of salt
- 2 tablespoons tomato sauce
- 3-4 tablespoons water
- 1/2 cup TVP, tofu or seitan
- 1/2 cup almond flour
- 1/2 teaspoon paprika
- 1/4 teaspoon oregano
- 1/4 cup cold margarine, cubed

Directions

1. Combine the almond flour, coconut flour, margarine, psyllium husk, and salt in a mixing dish. Make a crumbly dough using your hands (you can also do this in a food processor). Knead a bit more after adding the water. The dough may appear a little too moist at first, but as the flour absorbs the water, it will stiffen up. The dough should be divided into 8 little balls and placed in the fridge to rest for 5-10 minutes.

2. To make the filling, place the TVP in a small saucepan with just enough water to cover it. Combine the soy sauce and seasonings in a bowl. Bring to a boil, then reduce to low heat and continue to cook for about 5 minutes, or until the water has been absorbed. Allow it to cool somewhat before adding the tomato sauce.

3. Preheat the oven to 180 degrees Celsius (350

- 1/4 teaspoon ground cumin

degrees Fahrenheit). Remove the dough from the fridge and roll it out into 2 mm (a little less than 1/8 inch) round disks, keeping the dough from sticking with a cut-open ziplock bag. This is a nice time to utilize your tortilla press if you have one.

4. Place roughly a spoonful of filling in the center of a rolled-out piece of dough. To seal and form the empanada, fold the plastic over. Don't worry if it seems difficult at first; you'll get the hang of it. If the dough tears, just smooth out the cracks with your fingertips while gently stroking the plastic. Carefully pull the plastic off the formed empanada and lay it on a parchment-lined baking sheet.

5. Preheat the oven to 350°F and bake the empanadas for 12-15 minutes. Allow it to cool slightly before serving. They're delicious, both hot and cold. Serve with a fresh salad (non-starchy veggie of your choice) on the side.

Nutrition

Calories: 309 | Fat: 22.3g | Saturated Fat: 4.9g | Net Carbohydrates: 6.8g Protein: 11.5g | Fiber: 13.2g | Sugar: 1g | Sodium: 239mg

Keto Vegan Cauliflower Fried Rice With Tofu

Servings: 04

Preparation time: 10 minutes

Cook time: 20 minutes

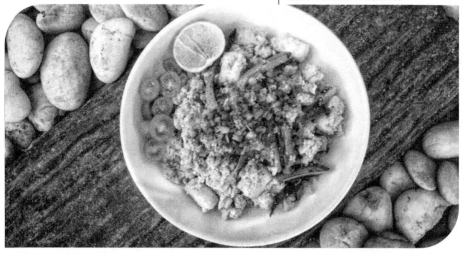

A well-balanced blend of seeds is the key to a creamy keto vegan porridge. In only a few minutes, you can cook a delicious keto vegan breakfast with this recipe.

Ingredients

- ½ tablespoon Kosher Salt
- 1/2 Green Onion
- 8-ounce Almond Flour
- ½ tablespoon Black Pepper
- 1 teaspoon Sesame Oil
- 1 tablespoon Olive Oil
- 4 tablespoons Less Sodium Soy Sauce
- 4 tablespoons Less Sodium Schezwan Sauce or Siracha sauce
- 1/4 cup vegetable broth
- 1 medium shredded cabbage
- 1 large shredded carrot
- 1/2 Red Onion

Directions

Marinate tofu and prepare vegetables:

1. Tofu should be cut into tiny squares and placed in a basin. On tofu, combine almond flour, soy sauce, salt, and Schezwan sauce (or Sriracha sauce). Allow it to marinate for at least 10 minutes.

2. The green onion should be coarsely chopped, and the onion should be thinly sliced. Also, create a coleslaw using cabbage and carrots that have been shredded.

Cook the cauliflower rice:

3. Heat the olive oil in a wok over medium heat. Stir in the cauliflower rice and season with salt to taste in the heated pan. Cook the rice until it begins to soften.

4. Follow the instructions on the back of the package if you're using packaged cauliflower rice.

5. Remove the rice from the wok and set it aside after it has finished cooking.

- 14-ounce block firm tofu, drained
- 1 medium head (16 oz.) Cauliflower Rice

Fry tofu:

6. In a skillet or wok, add a little extra olive oil and heat it up. In this pan, add the tofu pieces and lightly fry them over medium heat until they have a golden-brown crust.

7. Remove the tofu from the pan and set it aside on a platter. Allow it to rest for a while.

Fry vegetables and assemble:

8. In a wok, add the grated ginger and garlic. Maintain a high heat in the wok. Because the vegetables cook rapidly, make sure they're ready. Stir in the onions. After that, add the coleslaw and cook for a few minutes. Season with salt, black pepper, and other seasonings as desired. Stir in the soy sauce, vegetable broth, and Schezwan sauce for a few minutes until the sauces are well combined with the veggies.

9. In a mixing bowl, combine the fried cauliflower rice and tofu. And finally, add a teaspoon of sesame seed oil. Serve with chopped green onion and sesame seeds as a garnish.

Nutrition

Calories: 183 | Fat: 10.4g | Saturated Fat: 3.7g | Net Carbohydrates: 5.1g
Protein: 9.5g | Fiber: 4.2g | Sugar: 6.6g | Sodium: 325mg

Walnut Chili With Vegan Cheese And Sliced Avocado

Servings: 06

Preparation time: 10 minutes

Cook time: 30 minutes

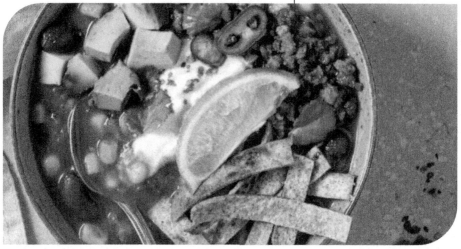

This vegan walnut chili, as the name implies, is loaded with walnuts, which are high in antioxidants and omega-3 fatty acids. Walnuts are also beneficial to brain function and digestive health. Enjoy this keto vegan walnut chili, knowing it's loaded with vitamins and minerals!

Ingredients

Chili:

- 5 medium celery stalks, diced
- 1 1/2 teaspoon ground cinnamon
- 5 tablespoon avocado oil
- 2 teaspoon chili powder
- 4 teaspoon cumin
- 1 1/2 teaspoon smoked paprika
- 15-ounce canned diced tomatoes
- 1 cup walnuts, crushed
- 2 medium green bell pepper, diced
- 2 teaspoon fresh garlic, minced

Directions

1. Heat the avocado oil in a skillet and add the celery. Cook, occasionally stirring, until softened, approximately 4-5 minutes.

2. Garlic, cinnamon, chili powder, cumin, and smoked paprika are added to the pan. Stir everything together until it's completely smooth.

3. Combine the bell pepper, zucchini, and mushrooms in a large mixing bowl. To taste, season with salt and pepper. Cook for a total of 4-6 minutes.

4. Combine the chipotle pepper, tomato paste, tomatoes, vegetable broth, coconut milk, vegan meat crumble or tempeh, walnuts, and unsweetened cocoa powder in a large mixing bowl. Stir until everything is completely combined. Allow 20-25 minutes for the chili to thicken and become spicy. If the chili is still too thin, add 2 tablespoons of

- 1 medium zucchini
- 4 cup vegetable broth
- 8-ounce cremini mushrooms
- 2-ounce chipotle peppers in adobo sauce
- 1/2 cup unsweetened carton coconut milk
- 20-ounce vegan meat crumbles or tempeh
- 1 tablespoon unsweetened cocoa powder
- 1 1/2 tablespoon tomato paste

Garnish:

- 1 cup vegan cheese
- 4 tablespoon red radish, sliced
- 4 tablespoon fresh cilantro
- Salt and pepper to taste
- 2 medium avocados, sliced

vegan cheese.

5. Fresh cilantro, avocado slices, sliced radishes, and vegan cheese go on top of the chili. To taste, season with more salt and pepper.

Nutrition

Calories: 533.2 | Fat: 35.4g | Saturated Fat: 5.3g | Net Carbohydrates: 5.8g
Protein: 29.9g | Fiber: 11.1g | Sugar: 7.3g | Sodium: 475mg

Cauliflower Crust Pizza Topped With Vegan Cheese

Servings: 01

Preparation time: 10 minutes

Cook time: 30 minutes

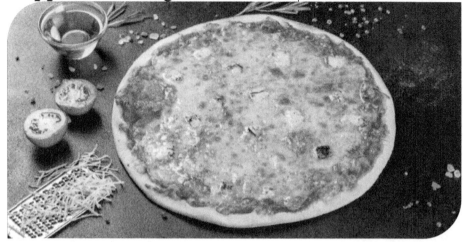

Because the fat content comes from the deliciously indulgent vegan cheese and almond flour, this Cauliflower Crust Pizza is ideal for keto vegan diets. It's also low in carbohydrates and high in delicious flavor.

Ingredients

- 4 oz Vegan cheese
- 1/4 cup water
- 1/3 cup almond flour
- 1 1/2 tsp baking powder or 2 1/2 tbsp ground flax or chia seeds
- 1/4 tsp garlic powder
- 1/2 medium head cauliflower (4 cups small florets)
- 1 tsp dried oregano, optional
- 1/2 tsp salt

Directions

1. Set aside a baking sheet lined with parchment paper. If using flax or chia seeds, combine them with the water and chill for at least half an hour. Cauliflower florets should be steamed until they are tender and fall apart. Drain completely. Combine the flour, oregano, garlic, salt, and baking powder in a mixing bowl (if using).

2. Preheat the oven to 450 degrees Fahrenheit. After the cauliflower has cooled slightly, press out as much liquid as possible with a clean dish towel or cheesecloth over a sink or basin. It should come out with at least 2/3 cup of water — you want it to be as dry as possible.

3. Pour the 1/4 cup water into a dish with the strained cauliflower (or the flax mixture). In a large mixing bowl, mash and whisk everything together thoroughly. Combine the flour and baking soda in a mixing bowl. Make a ball out of it. Arrange on a

baking sheet. Pat into a circle, then spread out with another sheet of parchment (and a rolling pin, if preferred) to approximately 1/4 inch thick.

4. Remove the top parchment sheet. Bake for 20 minutes, or until the edges are gently browned and crispy. Return to the oven and bake until the cheese is melted, adding toppings as desired. Bake for another 10 minutes. Allow 5 minutes for cooling. Cut and savor!

Nutrition

Calories: 61 | Fat: 3.7g | Saturated Fat: 0.4g | Net Carbohydrates: 1.7g
Protein: 2.8g | Fiber: 3.1g | Sugar: 1.4g | Sodium: 197.7mg

Eggplant Lasagna Made With Vegan Cheeses

Servings: 04

Preparation time: 15 minutes

Cook time: 35 minutes

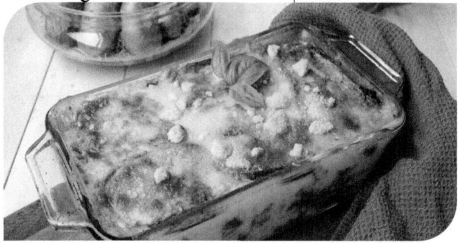

This Eggplant Lasagna is simple to make with few ingredients, inexpensive, and flavorful. This simple dish is an excellent choice for any quick family lunch. Because no one can tell it's vegan, it's made its way onto everyone's plates during ketogenesis.

Ingredients

- 1/4 cup olive oil
- 1 cup Vegan mozzarella, shredded
- 1 batch Vegan Parmesan Cheese (3 ingredients, 1 min)
- 2 batches Vegan Ricotta (Tofutti or Kite Hill)
- 2 cups Vegan marinara sauce
- 2 large eggplants, cut into slices
- 5 cloves garlic
- salt, pepper to taste

Optional:

- 2 tsp onion powder
- 4 tsp garlic powder
- 3 tsp Italian herbs

Directions

1. Preheat the oven to 410 degrees Fahrenheit and prepare a 10x10 casserole dish.

2. Begin by slicing the eggplants thinly. In a skillet, heat the olive oil and cook the eggplants for around 5 minutes. Set aside after seasoning with salt and pepper. Make sure the oil is really hot; this will give you a better texture and flavor. Make careful to drain any residual oil after cooking. Use a kitchen crêpe if necessary.

3. Then, in a bowl, combine marinara and garlic and season with a bit of salt and pepper. Combine the optional garlic powder, onion powder, and Italian herbs with the vegan ricotta that has been prepared.

4. Finally, get ready to layer your lasagna. Begin with a layer of marinara sauce on the bottom, then eggplants, vegan ricotta, marinara, and a pinch of

vegan Parmesan, followed by vegan mozzarella. Repeat till all of the materials have been utilized. Last but not least, a layer of marinara and ricotta, topped with Parmesan and Mozzarella.

5. Bake for 30 minutes, or until the vegan cheese has melted and become brown. Allow it to cool for about 5 to 8 minutes before serving.

Nutrition

Calories: 568.6 | Fat: 32.1g | Saturated Fat: 10.8g | Sodium: 389.3mg
Net Carbohydrates: 4.6g | Protein: 26.4g | Fiber: 11.1g | Sugar: 5.2g

Cauliflower Mac And Cheese

Servings: 04

Preparation time: 10 minutes

Cook time: 30 minutes

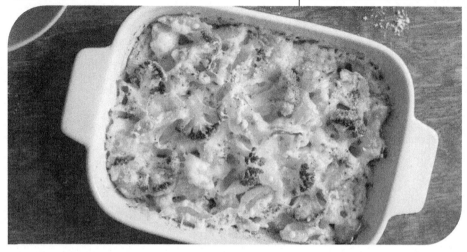

This recipe for cauliflower mac & cheese is a lot of fun and tasty! It's creamy and cozy, much like conventional mac and cheese, except instead of pasta, it's prepared with vegetables. It indicates that this cuisine is vegan, keto, and full of delicious tastes.

Ingredients

- For cauliflower base:
- 1 teaspoon olive oil
- 1/4 teaspoon sea salt
- 1 very large head of cauliflower or 2 small heads
- black pepper
- For cauliflower cashew cheese sauce:
- 3 tablespoons nutritional yeast
- 1 tablespoon fresh lemon juice
- 1 teaspoon Dijon mustard
- 1/3 cup hot water + more as needed
- 1/2 cup cashews, soaked in hot water

Directions

1. While the cauliflower is cooking, soak the cashews in boiling water for at least 30 minutes.

2. Cauliflower should be cut into bite-size pieces.

3. In a big, shallow pan, bring about 1/4 inch of water to a boil. Cauliflower florets with 1/4 teaspoon salt

4. Reduce heat to medium-high, cover, and cook for 6-8 minutes, or until fork-tender but not falling apart, stirring every 2 minutes or so.

5. Using a slotted spoon, remove all but 1 cup of cauliflower. Allow draining in a colander or on a towel-lined chopping board. Cook for another 3 minutes or until cauliflower is extremely tender and falling apart. If the water in the pan starts to evaporate too rapidly and the pan becomes dry, add extra water.

6. In a blender or food processor, combine the soft-cooked cup of cauliflower, soaked and drained cashews, nutritional yeast, lemon juice, mustard, garlic powder, turmeric, and sea salt, as well as the

100

- 1/2 teaspoon garlic powder
- 1/8 teaspoon turmeric
- 1 cup very soft cooked cauliflower
- 1 teaspoon sea salt
- For garnish:
- black pepper
- fresh herbs
- paprika

initial 1/3 cup of hot water. Blend on high speed until completely smooth, adding extra hot water if necessary. The final consistency should be pourable but not runny. I ended up adding just approximately 1 tablespoon more.

7. Clean the skillet you used to steam the cauliflower and put 1 tsp olive oil in it over medium heat. Return the drained cauliflower florets to the pan, along with 1/4 teaspoon salt and a few black pepper grinds. Stir in the olive oil, salt, and pepper to coat.

8. Pour the sauce over the cauliflower and toss lightly to coat. If necessary, season with additional salt. If using, season with cracked black pepper, paprika, and fresh herbs. Serve immediately, although it may be prepared ahead of time and simply reheated.

Nutrition

Calories: 185.4 | Fat: 10.2g | Saturated Fat: 3.4g | Net Carbohydrates: 3.8g
Protein: 9.2g | Fiber: 6g | Sugar: 4.8g | Sodium: 363.7mg

Keto Vegan Portobello Mushroom Burger

Servings: 02

Preparation time: 10 minutes

Cook time: 25 minutes

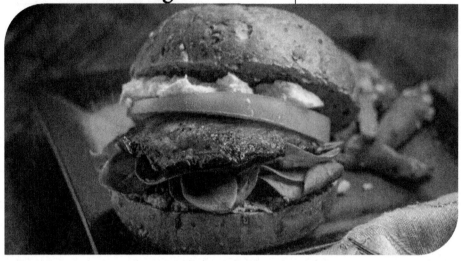

These keto vegan Portobello mushroom burgers are tasty and nutritious, making them ideal for a family get-together, a meal with friends, or a special treat after a hard day. They just call for a few ingredients, the majority of which are likely cupboard mainstays for many of you!

Ingredients

- 4 Portobello mushrooms
- 120 g plain tofu
- 1/2 medium-sized tomato
- 2 large salad leaves
- 3 tsp sugar-free mustard
- 2 1/2 tbsp olive oil
- 2 tbsp tamari (or soy sauce)
- a pinch of black pepper
- a pinch of ground cumin (optional)

Directions

1. One tablespoon tamari, 1 1/2 tablespoon olive oil, a dash of black pepper, and ground cumin combine the clean Portobello mushrooms. Use your hands to combine the ingredients, but be cautious with the mushrooms because they are prone to breaking. Now you can either saute the mushrooms right away or chill them for around 15 minutes.

2. Tofu should be cut into 2-4 thick pieces. To make the tofu marinade, use 1 tablespoon of olive oil instead of 2 1/2 tablespoons. You may either cook it right away or let it rest in the fridge for about 20 minutes.

3. Wash and chop the remaining veggies for the recipe according to your tastes.

4. In a preheated oven at 180°C, bake the mushrooms for 10-15 minutes. Turn them a couple of times to keep them from drying out too much. Keep the

oven door open for the final 5 minutes to ensure that the cooked mushrooms are tender but not watery.

5. Tofu and mushrooms may be baked together. Cook for 8-10 minutes to keep the tofu supple or until browned for a crispy finish.

6. Assemble the burgers while the mushrooms and tofu are still warm and serve right away. Although you may prepare the ingredients ahead of time, it's best to assemble the burgers right before serving.

Nutrition

Calories: 255.1 | Fat: 20.7g | Saturated Fat: 4.8g | Net Carbohydrates: 6.8g
Protein: 11g | Fiber: 4.1g | Sugar: 0.8g | Sodium: 25.4mg

Keto Vegan Bibimbap

Servings: 02

Preparation time: 15 minutes

Cook time: 10 minutes

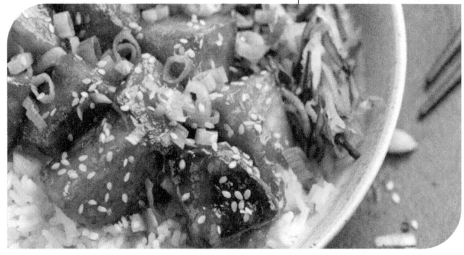

This is a good quick-filling meal that takes around half an hour to cook and has a variety of tastes. If you can't locate gochujang, use sriracha in this recipe, along with a dash of miso for the fermented ingredient. It will have a little different flavor, but it will still be excellent.

Ingredients

- 200 g / 7 oz tempeh, sliced into squares
- 4-6 broccoli florets, in thin spears
- 1 carrot, grated
- 1/2 cucumber, in strips
- 1 tablespoon soy sauce
- 300 g / 10 oz raw cauliflower, riced
- 2 tablespoons gochujang chili paste (or sriracha)
- 2 tablespoons rice vinegar (or regular white)
- 2 tablespoons rice vinegar (or regular white vinegar)

Directions

1. In a dish, combine the soy sauce and vinegar, then dip the tempeh squares in it. Set them away for a few moments.

2. Meanwhile, prepare your vegetables. Heat some oil in a pan and sauté the tempeh over medium heat. When it's done, remove it from the pan. Continue to cook the peppers, broccoli, and carrots in the same pan.

3. Cover and simmer for a minute or two to retain some of the bites of the vegetables. In a separate pan, stir cook the cauliflower rice with a little oil until tender.

4. Combine the chili paste, vinegar, soy sauce, oil, and sweetener in a small bowl. If the sauce is too thick, thin it up with a little water. Place the tempeh, peppers, broccoli, carrot, and raw cucumber on top

104

- 1 tablespoon soy sauce
- 1 teaspoon sesame oil
- 1 small red bell pepper, in strips
- concentrated liquid sweetener to taste
- 2 tablespoons sesame seeds

of the cauliflower rice on two plates.

5. Drizzle the chili sauce over the vegetables and tempeh, then top with sesame seeds. Before serving or eating, combine everything on your dish.

Nutrition

Calories: 229 | Fat: 12.4g | Saturated Fat: 3.7g | Net Carbohydrates: 8.9g
Protein: 18.3g | Fiber: 8.7g | Sugar: 1.6g | Sodium: 339mg

Keto Vegan Seitan Negimaki

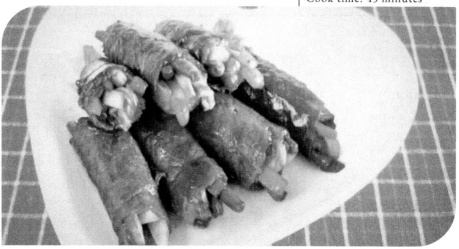

Seitan is beautifully cooked teriyaki buns packed with vivid scallions. The simple marinade of hoisin and mirin does an excellent job of keeping the meat moist while providing the proper balance of sweet and salty flavors.

Ingredients

For the simmering broth:

- 8 cups vegetable broth
- 6 cloves garlic, smashed
- 1/4 cup fresh sliced ginger

For the seitan:

- 1 1/4 cups vital wheat gluten
- 3 tablespoons nutritional yeast flakes
- 3/4 cup cold water
- 1/4 cup soy sauce

For the marinade:

- 1/3 cup hoisin sauce
- 1/4 cup mirin
- 3 tablespoons water
- 2 teaspoons Sriracha

Directions

Make the seitan:

1. In a large saucepan, combine all of the ingredients for the simmering broth and bring to a boil. Meanwhile, prepare the seitan.

2. In a mixing dish, combine wheat gluten and nutritional yeast. Knead in the water and soy sauce for two to three minutes, or until a firm dough forms.

3. Make a flat log out of the dough that is about 8 inches long and 4 inches wide.

4. Lower the heat to a low simmer and immerse the seitan after the soup has reached a boil. Cook for 30 minutes with the lid ajar to allow steam to escape. Allow the broth to cool fully before serving.

Marinade:

5. Begin the marinade after the seitan has cooled. In a wide, shallow bowl, combine all of the ingredients.

6. Slice the seitan now. It should be approximately an

106

(plus extra for garnish)

- 1 teaspoon fresh ginger, micro planed or minced to a paste
- 1 teaspoon toasted sesame oil

Dressing:

- 2 bunches scallions, green parts only, sliced 3 to 4 inches long
- A few tablespoons of toasted sesame seeds
- Plain wooden toothpicks

eighth of an inch thick, but it doesn't have to be precisely even. Just make sure the slice is long enough to wrap around your pinky without breaking or becoming unmanageable.

7. Place the 16 slices in the marinade for an hour, turning them halfway through.

Assemble and cook:

8. Move all of the seitan to the side of the marinade dish and add the cut scallions, covering them with sauce. So, roughly, one side seitan and one side scallion should be in your dish.

9. To avoid a mess, form the rolls on a dinner plate. Place a thin slice of marinated seitan on a dinner platter. Place 4 or 5 scallions across, with an inch or two of scallions sticking out the ends. Roll the seitan around the scallion, securing it with toothpicks if necessary. Make sure the toothpicks are all going in the same direction so you can grill them without them getting in the way.

10. Heat the grill over medium heat after the rolls are made. Cook rolls until grill marks emerge, spraying or brushing the grill with oil. On my indoor cast iron grill, I did 8 at a time, and it took around 4 minutes. To turn the rolls, use a metal spatula to reach underneath them and spray extra oil as needed. Cook until grill marks emerge on the opposite side.

11. Place the buns on a serving platter. When ready to serve, drizzle with remaining marinade and sriracha (or leave it out if you don't like it hot) and top with toasted sesame seeds. Serve!

Nutrition

Calories: 299.1 | Fat: 6.2g | Saturated Fat: 0.4g | Net Carbohydrates: 8.8g
Protein: 31g | Fiber: 5.5g | Sugar: 2.9g | Sodium: 387.8mg

Keto Vegan Nut Bars

Bars: 10

Preparation time: 10 minutes

Chill: 1 hour

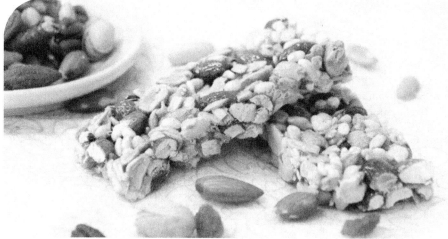

This simple snack is low in carbs, high in fat, and free of eggs, making it a terrific freezer-friendly keto vegan snack to grab and go! These bars will satisfy your sweet cravings at any time of day with only 8 ingredients and a short prep time.

Ingredients

- 1/2 cup desiccated coconut
- 1/4 teaspoon salt
- 1/3 cup Sukrin Gold Fiber Syrup See link
- 2 tablespoons coconut oil or butter
- 2 cups Mixed nuts and seeds
- 1 teaspoon vanilla essence
- 3 tablespoons almond butter or peanut butter
- 1 tablespoon chia seeds

Directions

1. Using the baking paper, line a 20cm square baking pan. If necessary, gently oil it to aid in the sticking of the paper.

2. Chop the bigger nuts coarsely. You may leave them whole, but the bar will be crumblier. Combine the desiccated coconut, chia seeds, and salt in a large mixing dish.

3. Combine the coconut oil/butter, vanilla, almond butter, and fiber syrup in a small microwave-safe bowl.

4. Microwave the oil and butter combination for 30 seconds or until it readily mixes. To ensure that everything is uniformly mixed, stir everything together thoroughly.

5. Pour the melted mixture over the nuts and seeds and stir to blend completely.

6. Use the back of a measuring cup to press the

mixture into the baking tray firmly and evenly.

7.   Refrigerate for 1 hour before cutting, or freeze until ready to eat.

Nutrition

Calories: 271.4 | Fat: 22g | Saturated Fat: 4g | Net Carbohydrates: 7.7g
Protein: 7.1g | Fiber: 11.2g | Sugar: 1.1g | Sodium: 63mg

Keto Vegan Coconut Fat Bombs

Bombs: 18

Preparation time: 10 minutes

Chill: 1 hour

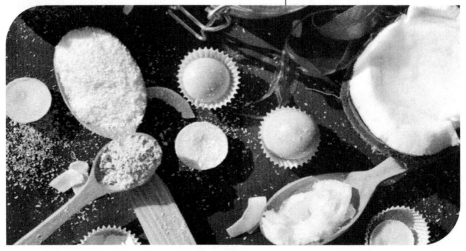

With only 4 ingredients, you can make these nutritious keto vegan Coconut Fat Bombs in no time! The coconut taste is bursting at the seams. These Coconut Fat Bombs are for you if you want to add extra coconut oil to your diet or if you're on a keto vegan diet. A delicious low-carb summer treat that also makes a great edible gift!

Ingredients

- ½ cup coconut butter, melted
- ½ cup coconut oil, melted
- ¼ cup + 2 tablespoons finely shredded coconut
- 12 drops stevia

Directions

1. Combine all of the ingredients. Fill tiny cupcake liners or an ice cube tray with 1 tbsp each using a tablespoon.

2. Freeze for 1 hour. Place in the refrigerator.

Nutrition

Calories: 93.5 | Fat: 9.1g | Saturated Fat: 5.8g | Net Carbohydrates: 1.6g
Protein: 1g | Fiber: 1g | Sugar: 0.2g | Sodium: 1.4mg

Spicy Roasted Peanuts

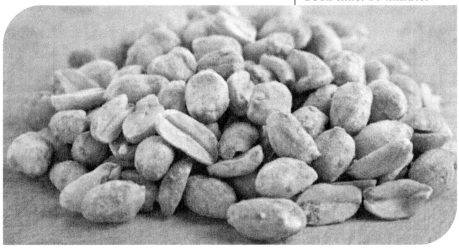

Make your own roasted nuts at home for a low-carb vegan snack that's quick and easy! This recipe asks for an air fryer to make spicy peanuts, which may be roasted in any oil of your choice. Season to taste and/or add additional nuts of your choosing!

Ingredients

- 2 Tbsp. Olive Oil
- 2 cups Raw Peanuts, unshelled
- 2 tsp. Old Bay Seasoning
- ½ tsp. Sea Salt
- ¼ tsp. Cayenne Pepper
- 1 Tbsp. Nutritional Yeast
- 2 tsp. Cholula Hot Sauce

Directions

1. Set aside a baking sheet lined with parchment paper.

2. In a mixing dish, combine all of the ingredients and swirl to fully coat the peanuts.

3. Fill the air fryer halfway with the nut mixture and distribute the peanuts out evenly.

4. Air fried for 10 minutes at 330 degrees.

5. To cool, pour the peanuts onto a baking sheet lined with parchment paper.

6. Allow the nuts to cool completely before transferring them to a sealed container or bag.

Nutrition

Calories: 243 | Fat: 22g | Saturated Fat: 4.4g | Net Carbohydrates: 2.7g
Protein: 9.3g | Fiber: 3.4g | Sugar: 2.1g | Sodium: 164mg

Keto Vegan Celery Snacks

Servings: 16
Preparation time: 10 minutes
Cook time: 0 minutes

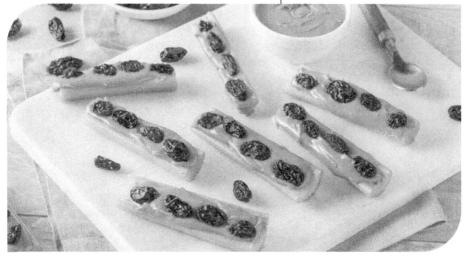

Made with few ingredients, this dish is easy and tasty. Every bite is filled with creamy richness, making this a snack to look forward to.

Ingredients

- 1 lb. (16 oz) celery
- 1-2 tbsp vegan cream cheese
- a sprinkle of everything bagel seasoning (per celery)
- 1-2 tbsp peanut butter or almond butter
- a few sugar-free chocolate chips (per celery)

Directions

1. Trim and discard the celery tops after removing the celery root. After cleaning and rinsing the stalks, split them in half.

2. Fill each stalk with cream cheese or peanut butter, then top with your favorite toppings.

3. I sprinkle everything bagel spice on the cream cheese-filled ones and vegan sugar-free chocolate chips on the peanut butter-filled ones.

4. It's time to eat.

Nutrition

Calories: 95 | Fat: 7g | Saturated Fat: 3.8g | Net Carbohydrates: 1.1g
Protein: 3g | Fiber: 1.6g | Sugar: 2.7g | Sodium: 143.4mg

Strawberry Muffins

Servings: 12

Preparation time: 10 minutes

Cook time: 12 minutes

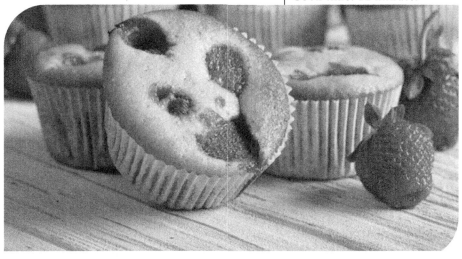

Strawberry muffins are low-carb and healthy, making them ideal for a keto vegan or gluten-free diet. They're ideal for a quick and tasty light snack. They're especially delicious when strawberries are in season.

Ingredients

- 3 tbsp flaxseeds grinded
- 6 tbsp water
- 2 cups almond flour
- 2 tsp baking powder
- 1/2 cup plant-based milk
- 1/3 cup coconut oil melted
- 1 tbsp vanilla extract
- 1/4 cup liquid sweetener stevia, erythritol, or monk fruit
- 1 1/4 cup fresh strawberries diced

Directions

1. Preheat the oven to 180 degrees Celsius (356 degrees Fahrenheit).

2. Combine flaxseeds and water in a small cup or bowl and set aside for a few minutes.

3. Combine almond flour and baking powder in a separate large mixing dish. Combine the coconut oil, milk, vanilla extract, and liquid sweetener in a mixing bowl. Stir everything together thoroughly.

4. Add the flaxseed mixture that has been produced. Use a wooden spatula to combine the ingredients.

5. Fold in the diced strawberries gently.

6. In a nonstick muffin pan, place the muffin paper cups. Fill each paper cup halfway with muffin batter. Bake for 12 minutes, or until a

wooden stick inserted into the center comes out clean.

Nutrition

Calories: 191.3 | Fat: 16.7g | Saturated Fat: 5.2g | Net Carbohydrates: 4.7g
Protein: 5.3g | Fiber: 3.1g | Sugar: 1.7g | Sodium: 87.6mg

Baked Kale Chips

Servings: 04

Preparation time: 5 minutes

Cook time: 25 minutes

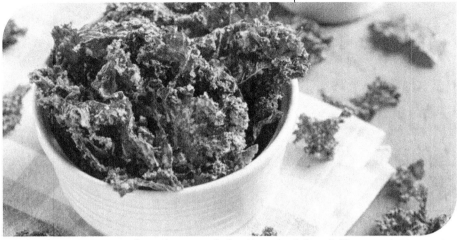

With a basic version, salt and vinegar kale chips, and five different spice varieties, this baked kale chips recipe are amazingly simple.

Ingredients

- 5 oz Kale (cut into pieces, stems removed)
- 1 tbsp Olive oil
- 1 tbsp White vinegar
- 3 tbsp Nutritional yeast (divided)
- 1/4 tsp Sea salt

Directions

1. Preheat oven to 300 degrees Fahrenheit (149 degrees C). Use parchment paper or silicone mats to line two baking sheets.

2. Whisk together the olive oil and white vinegar in a large mixing dish. Add the kale pieces to the oil and vinegar mixture and massage it into the kale.

3. 2/3 of the nutritional yeast and all of the sea salt should be combined. To uniformly scatter the ingredients, mix them together. Arrange the cookies on the baking sheets in a single layer. Top with the leftover nutritional yeast.

4. Bake for 20-25 minutes, until crispy, turning the pans halfway through.

Nutrition

Calories: 71 | Fat: 4.4g | Saturated Fat: 0.8g | Net Carbohydrates: 2.9g
Protein: 4.7g | Fiber: 1.6g | Sugar: 0.3g | Sodium: 25mg

Coconut Clusters

Balls: 15

Preparation time: 5 minutes

Cook time: 15 minutes

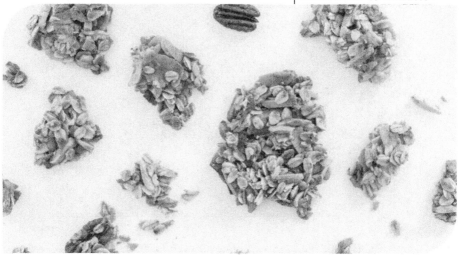

Coconut and seed balls create a delicious keto vegan snack. Once you tried it, you won't forget.

Ingredients

- 1 ½ cups coconut chips or desiccated, unsweetened
- ¼ cup chia seeds
- ¼ cup hemp seeds
- ½ cup pumpkin seeds
- 2 tables liquid monk fruit sweetener or another liquid sweetener

Directions

1. Combine all of the ingredients in a medium mixing basin and stir thoroughly.

2. The mixture should be spooned into walnut-sized forms and slightly squeezed to hold a shape. Place the clusters on a tray lined with parchment paper.

3. Preheat oven to 180°C/350°F and bake for 15 minutes.

4. Allow the clusters to cool before removing them from the tray. Put them in the fridge to solidify since they are brittle.

Nutrition

Calories: 75.3 | Fat: 6.5g | Saturated Fat: 1.6g | Net Carbohydrates: 3.1g
Protein: 3.5g | Fiber: 2.2g | Sugar: 1g | Sodium: 5.1mg

CONCLUSION

A keto vegan diet consists of a very low carbohydrate, high-fat, moderate-protein diet that excludes animal products. Weight loss and a decreased risk of heart disease and diabetes are related to both vegan and ketogenic diets.

It is, however, an extremely rigid diet that is not appropriate for everyone. The diet comes with a number of drawbacks, including the chance of nutritional deficiency. In the early stages, some people may experience side effects such as headaches and weariness.

Non-starchy veggies, avocados, nuts, seeds, coconut, vegan protein sources, and healthy oils are all keto vegan diet staples.

When following a keto vegan diet, limit animal products as well as high-carbohydrate items like grains, sugary drinks, and starchy vegetables.

When following a keto vegan diet, there are many wonderful items to pick from. The recipes provided in this book has meals and snacks that are high in healthy fats and low in carbohydrates.

To prevent deficiencies, it's important to properly prepare a keto vegan diet and take nutritional supplements. Pregnant women, children, and persons with certain medical issues may not be able to follow a low-carb, high-fat diet. If you're not sure if the keto vegan diet is good for you, consult your doctor about it.

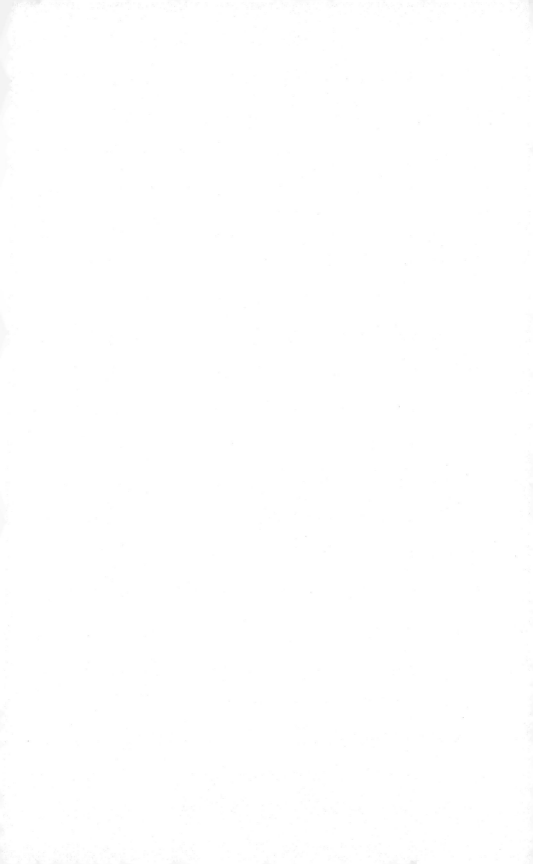

Printed in Great Britain
by Amazon